DIAGNOSTIC PICTURE TESTS IN

GERIATRIC MEDICINE

W9-AXE-396

ASIF KAMAL
FRCP (Lond)
Consultant Physician in Geriatric Medicine
St George's Hospital, Lincoln

Wolfe Medical Publications Ltd

Copyright © A. Kamal 1990
Published in 1990 by Wolfe Medical Publications Ltd
Reprinted 1992 by BPCC Hazells Ltd, Aylesbury, England
ISBN 0 7234 1565 X

For a full list of Wolfe Medical Atlases, plus
forthcoming titles and details of our surgical,
dental and veterinary Atlases, please write to
Wolfe Medical Publications Limited,
2-16 Torrington Place,
London WC1E 7LT

A CIP catalogue record for this book
is available from the British Library.

Preface

Clinical presentation of disease in old age is often unique, and usually different from similar conditions in younger patients. Together with the fact that elderly patients also show changes of ageing and of multiple pathology, this tends to make accurate clinical assessment both challenging and at times difficult. This is one reason why this speciality has a special status within the field of general medicine. The range of illustrations in this volume is as broad as possible, reflecting the great variety of signs seen in geriatric medicine.

This book is intended for all medical and paramedical personnel who are involved in the clinical management of elderly patients - especially undergraduate and postgraduate medical students, junior hospital doctors and general practitioners. It should be used as a tool for revising the clinical aspects of medicine in old age. It should also be of value to those preparing for examinations, particularly the MRCP exams and Diploma in Geriatric Medicine.

The answers to the questions are given as general guidelines and should serve as useful starting points for further discussion.

A. Kamal
Lincoln

Author's acknowledgements

My thanks to Dr Simon Leach for providing illustrations **9** and **149**, to Dr T. Powell for **16, 21, 42, 52, 113, 127, 152, 156**, to Dr Leeming for **29**, to Mr Lamerton for **34**, to Dr Scott for **48** and **106**, to Dr Prangnell for **68, 118, 139, 170** and to Boehringer Ingelheim Ltd for **81, 169** and **182**.

My special thanks to Glenise de Lacy for typing the manuscript and to the Department of Medical Illustrations at St George's Hospital, Lincoln, for taking many of the pictures in this volume.

1 This elderly patient was admitted with pain and swelling in the right leg. She gave past medical history of right knee replacement.
(a) Give two likely diagnoses.
(b) What complications may occur in this case?

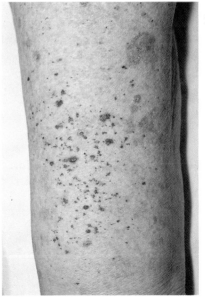

2 (a) Give four causes of this condition.
(b) What investigations are indicated?

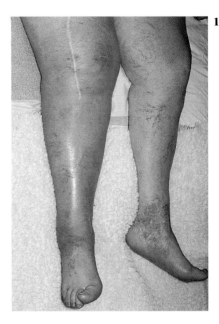

3 This 80 year old patient has a painful mouth.
(a) What is the diagnosis?
(b) What may be the underlying condition?

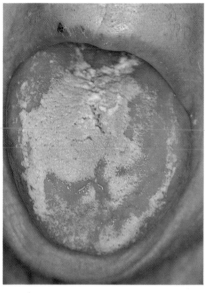

4 This elderly man underwent below knee amputation for severe peripheral vascular disease.
(a) What are the main elements of post-operative rehabilitation?
(b) What long term problems might occur in this patient?

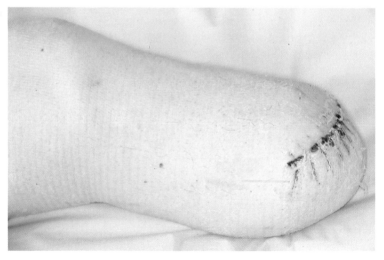

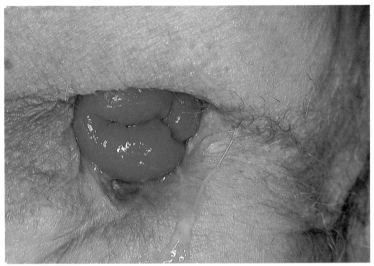

5 (a) What is this condition?
(b) What complications might occur?

6 This elderly man was admitted with a history of headaches and hypertension.
(a) What diagnosis is suggested by the facial appearance?
(b) What are the causes of this syndrome?

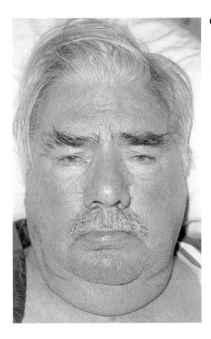

7

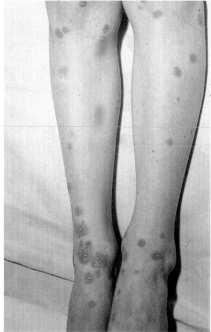

7 (a) What is this skin condition?
(b) What are the clinical features of Stevens-Johnson syndrome?

8

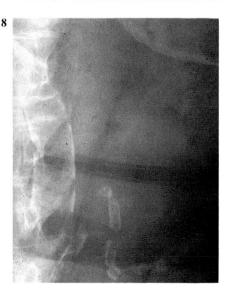

8 (a) What abnormality is seen in this plain X-ray of the abdomen?
(b) Are further investigations necessary?

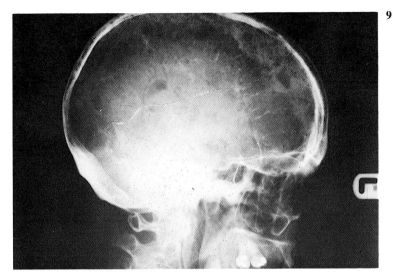

9 (a) What investigations are necessary after seeing this skull X-ray?
(b) What problems may this patient experience?

10 (a) What is this condition?
(b) Which investigations are required?

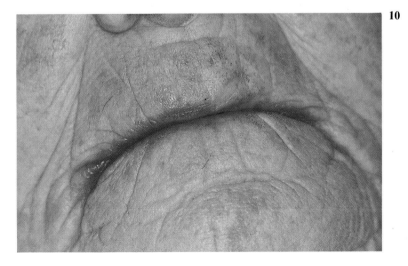

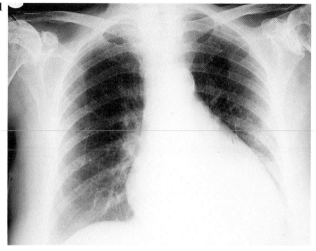

11 This chest X-ray is of a 70 year old patient who complains of dyspnoea on exertion of long standing and has suffered one minor stroke.
(a) What are the typical auscultatory findings in such cases?
(b) Name the complications that can occur in this patient?

12 (a) Identify the abnormalities seen in this hand.
(b) What are the special features of this disorder in the elderly?

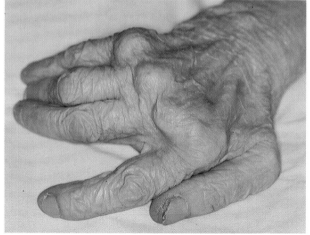

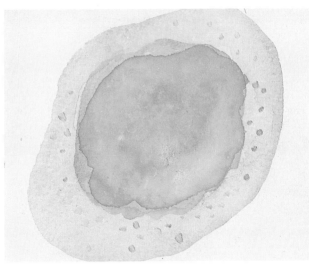

13 An erythroblast from the bone marrow of an 80 year old with anaemia.
(a) Which drugs can cause this type of anaemia?
(b) Describe the typical features of this anaemia.

14 This skin condition was seen in a 90 year old patient.
(a) What does this condition tell us about the woman's living conditions?
(b) Which investigations are necessary?

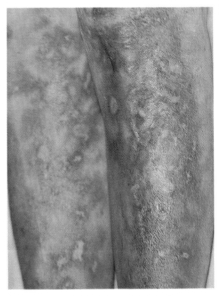

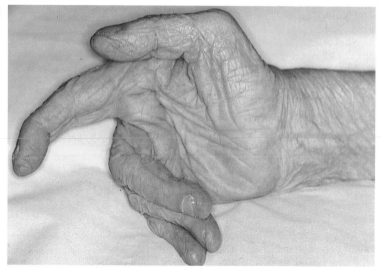

15 (a) What is this condition?
(b) Which disorders are associated with this abnormality?
(c) What is the preferred surgical treatment?

16 (a) Describe the clinical features which may be present in this patient.
(b) How should this case be managed?

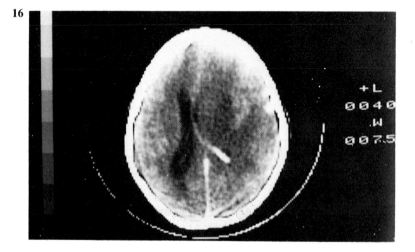

17 This elderly patient has chronic oedema of the feet.
(a) What are the likely causes?
(b) What are the common side-effects of diuretics used to treat such cases?

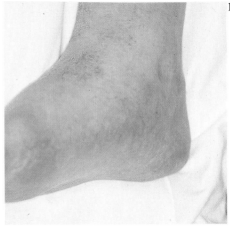

18 (a) What is this condition called?
(b) What symptoms may be present in this patient?

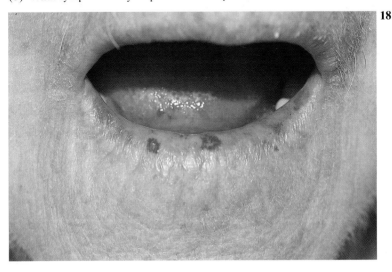

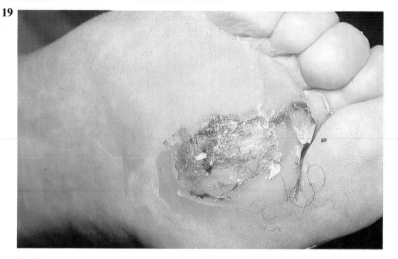

19 This 75 year old woman was admitted with recurrent falls.
(a) What is the most likely cause of her falls?
(b) What are the commonest environmental causes of recurrent falls in old age?

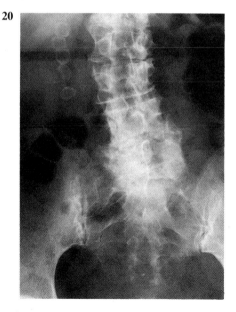

20 (a) What symptoms might this patient have?
(b) What are the different types of gall stones seen in elderly people?

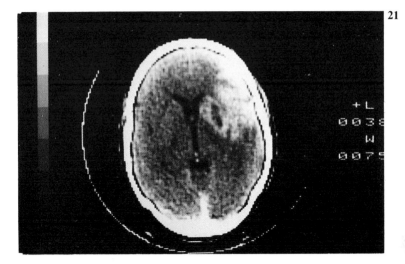

21 This patient presented with sudden collapse and unconsciousness.
(a) What does the CT scan show?
(b) Which neurological signs may be present?

22 (a) What symptoms might this patient have?
(b) What are the causes of hypercalcaemia in the elderly?

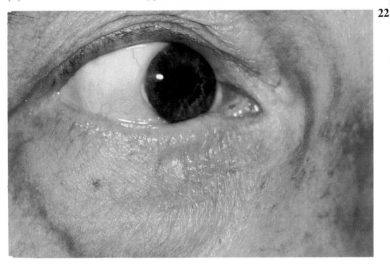

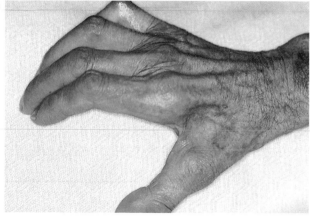

23 (a) What is wrong with this hand?
(b) What are the causes of this deformity?

24 A histological picture of cardiac muscle biopsy from an elderly man.
(a) What does it show?
(b) How does this condition present?

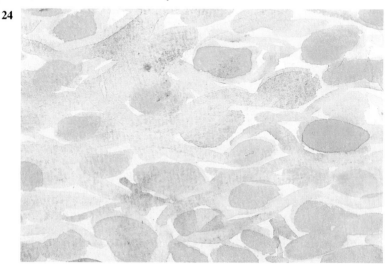

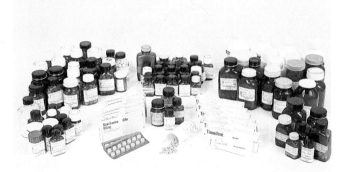

25 This collection of drugs was found in the kitchen of an elderly patient who was admitted to hospital with confusion, falls and incontinence.
(a) What are the major causes of adverse drug reactions in the elderly?
(b) Which measures may help in improving patient compliance?

26 This elderly lady presented with increasing lethargy, weight gain and bradycardia.
(a) What is the most likely diagnosis?
(b) What complications may occur?
(c) What is the treatment?

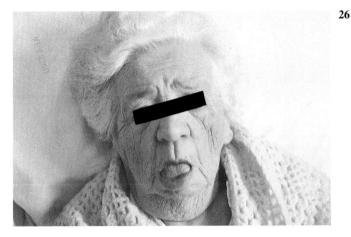

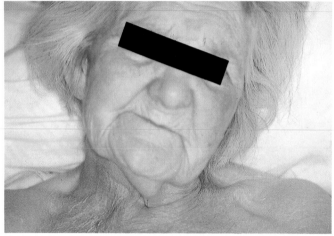

27 (a) What abnormality is seen in the neck?
(b) Which conditions are associated with this disorder?

28 This obese elderly lady presented with intense irritation around the genital area.
(a) What is the likely diagnosis?
(b) Which drugs can be used to treat this condition?
(c) What underlying conditions need to be excluded in this patient?

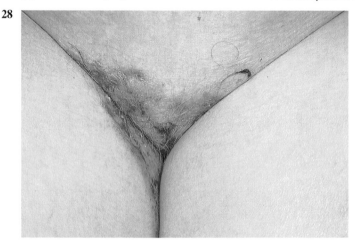

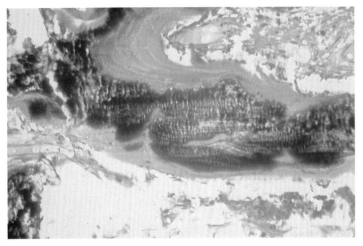

29 This histological picture is from a bone biopsy taken from an elderly patient.
(a) What does it show?
(b) Describe the clinical features of this patient.
(c) What is the diagnostic radiological feature?

30 (a) What abnormality is seen in this X-ray?
(b) What biochemical abnormalities may be associated with this condition?

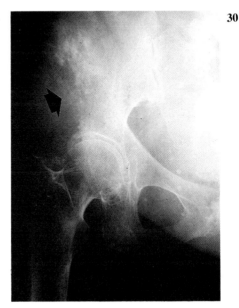

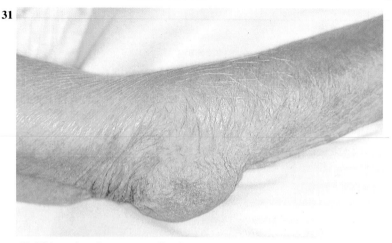

31 This patient has a generalized systemic disorder.
(a) What abnormality is seen in the elbow?
(b) Name other periarticular soft tissue manifestations which may be present in this case.

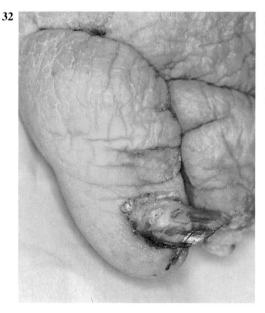

32 (a) What is this condition called?
(b) Which patients are prone to this disorder?
(c) Name six common abnormalities seen in the feet of elderly patients.

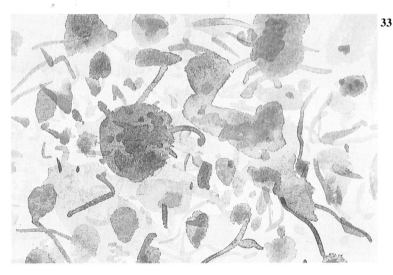

33 This picture is from brain tissue histology of an elderly man.
(a) What does it show?
(b) Which other histological features are usually present in such cases?

34 This arteriogram was performed in an elderly man.
(a) Describe the abnormalities.
(b) What would this patient complain of?

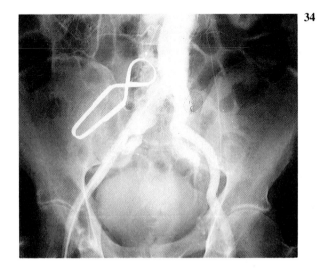

35

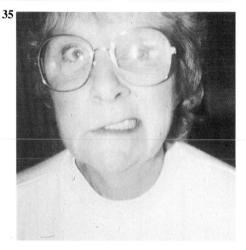

35 This lady developed sudden right facial palsy.
(a) What other problems may be present in this case?
(b) What are the main types of paralysis of the facial muscles?

36

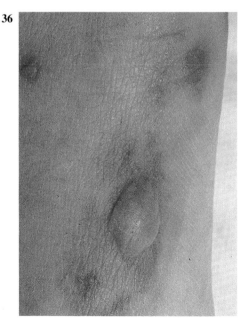

36 This elderly patient presented with a long history of persistent burning pruritus.
(a) What does the picture show?
(b) What sites are typically affected?
(c) What is this condition associated with?

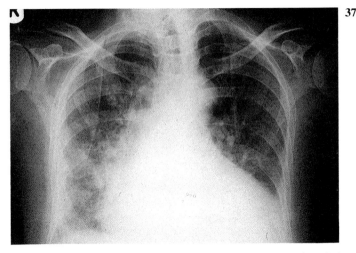

37 This X-ray is of an elderly patient who was admitted to hospital as an emergency.
(a) What symptoms did she have?
(b) What are the causes of this condition in the elderly?

38 This elderly man has severe pain in the big toe.
(a) Which investigations should be done?
(b) What is the treatment?

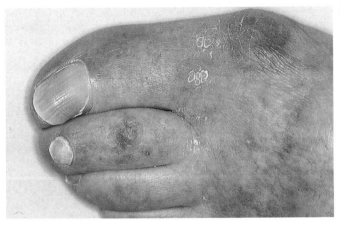

39

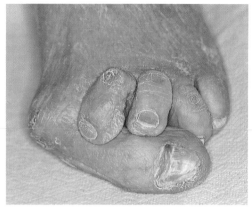

39 (a) Describe this condition.
(b) What problems might the patient have?

40 (a) Describe what is happening here.
(b) Which problems might occur during this stage of rehabilitation?

40

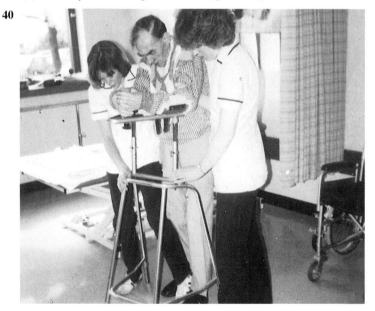

41 This elderly patient has chronic oedema of the feet.
(a) Give four common causes.
(b) Which drugs can cause peripheral oedema?

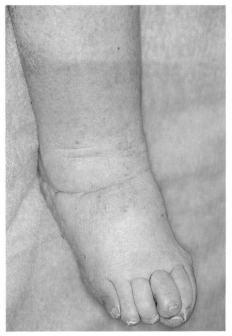

42 (a) What does this CT scan show?
(b) What symptoms might the patient have?
(c) What signs may be present?

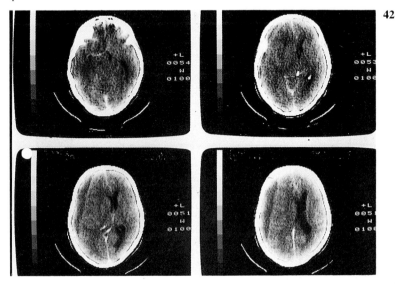

43

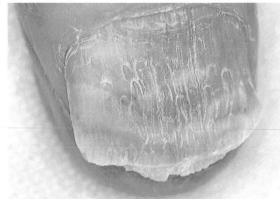

43 (a) Describe this finger nail.
(b) What abnormalities may be seen in the blood count and indices?
(c) This patient also had dysphagia. What is the diagnosis?

44 X-ray of the pelvis of an 80 year old woman.
(a) What abnormality is shown?
(b) What are the other causes of pelvic calcification in an elderly patient?

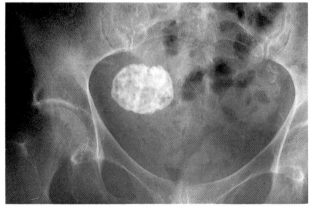

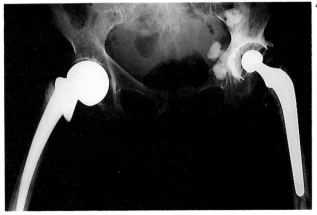

45 This 75 year old patient has had bilateral hip operations for fractures of the neck of femurs resulting from minor trauma.
(a) What bone abnormality would you expect to see?
(b) What general complications may occur in an elderly patient following surgery for hip repair?

46 Chest X-ray showing features of chronic bronchitis in a 68 year old patient.
(a) What organisms are most commonly seen in the sputum during an acute exacerbation?
(b) What will the pulmonary function tests reveal?

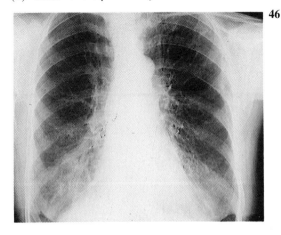

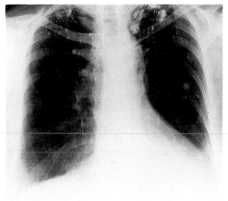

47 This patient presented with history of cough, dyspnoea, weight loss, anorexia and excessive sweating.
(a) What does the chest X-ray show?
(b) What condition needs to be excluded?
(c) Give three causes of pulmonary calcification.

48 (a) What does this gastroscopy show?
(b) What are the clinical features of this condition?

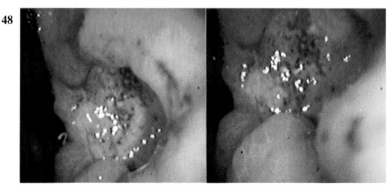

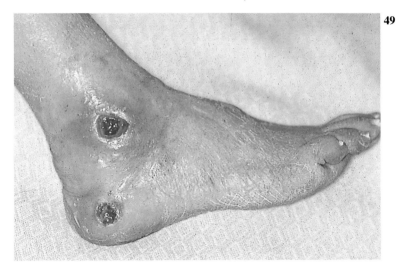

49 (a) What is the most likely cause of this perforating ulceration?
(b) What other dermatological complications may be seen in such cases?

50 (a) Which drugs can cause this condition?
(b) What other disorders is this condition associated with?

51

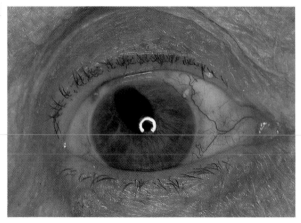

51 (a) What is this pupillary abnormality due to?
(b) What are the other causes of pupillary abnormalities in the elderly?

52 This elderly man presented with increasing forgetfulness, odd behaviour and nocturnal agitation.
(a) What does the CT scan show?
(b) What is the most likely diagnosis?
(c) Which organic brain disorders can present with an identical clinical picture?

52

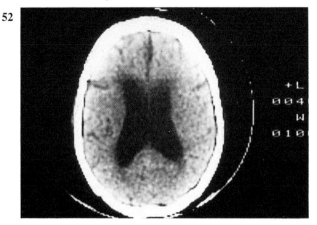

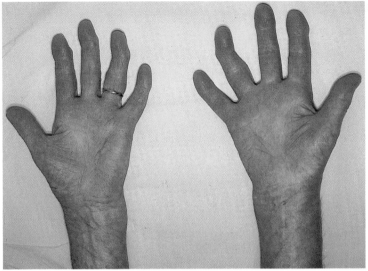

53 (a) What other skin signs would you look for in this patient?
(b) What complications may occur in this case?

54 (a) What clinical features are shown in this barium enema X-ray?
(b) Are there any aetiological factors?

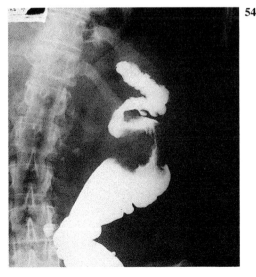

55

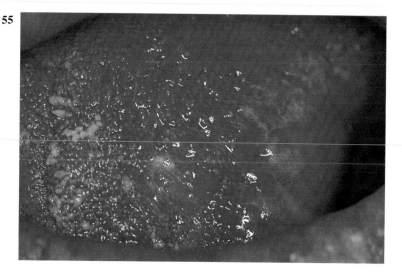

55 (a) What is the diagnosis?
(b) What are the likely underlying causes of this condition?

56

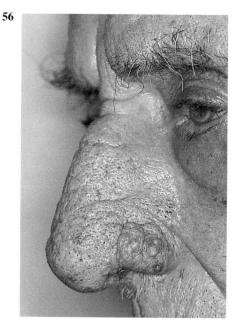

56 (a) What is the diagnosis?
(b) Which skin condition is this disorder associated with?
(c) What is the pathology?

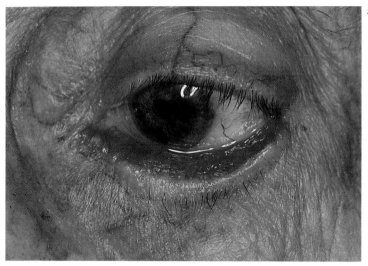

57 This is a common ocular disorder in the elderly.
(a) What is it?
(b) What is the treatment?

58 (a) What features are seen in this X-ray of the knee?
(b) What problems does this condition cause in elderly patients?
(c) What abnormalities will be seen in synovial biopsy?

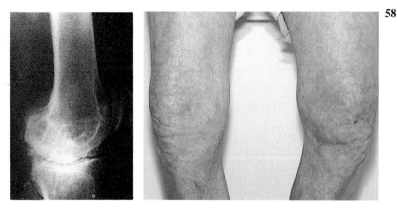

59

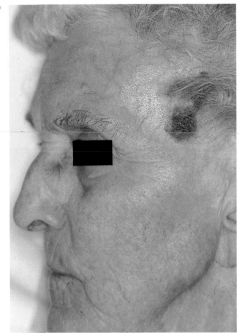

59 (a) What is this lesion called?
(b) What is the differential diagnosis?

60 This elderly patient presented with recurrent faints.
(a) What does the ECG show?
(b) What is the treatment of this condition?

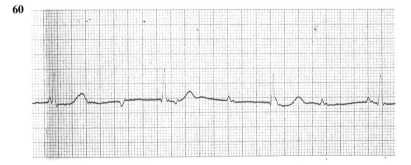

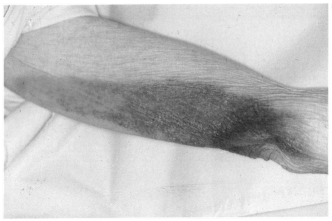

61 This 85 year old, who lived alone in a state of neglect and malnutrition, presented with extensive non-traumatic bruising on her arms and legs.
(a) Give the three most likely causes of her bruising.
(b) What are the features of hypovitaminosis-C in the elderly?

62 (a) What is this common condition?
(b) How is it formed?

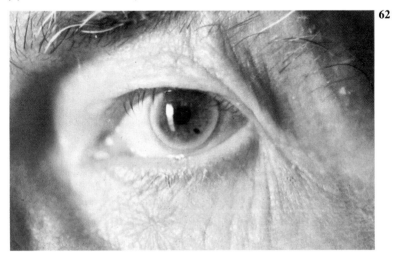

63 (a) What does this chest X-ray show?
(b) What are the likely causes of this abnormality in an elderly patient?

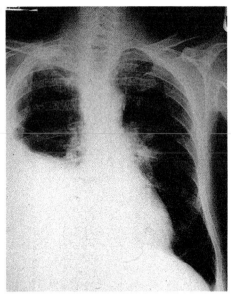

64 (a) What abnormality is seen in this fundus?
(b) What is the classical symptom accompanying this abnormality?
(c) What other features may be present in such cases?

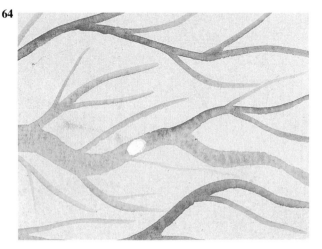

65 (a) What is this lesion?
(b) Which factors are
important in its aetiology?

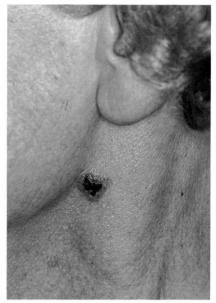

66 This 78 year old presented with lethargy,
depression and obesity.
(a) What does the ECG show?
(b) What is the likely underlying diagnosis?
(c) What other cardiac abnormalities may occur in
this condition?

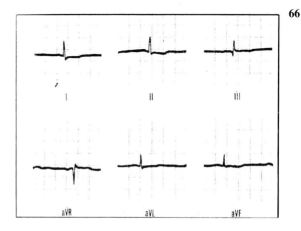

67

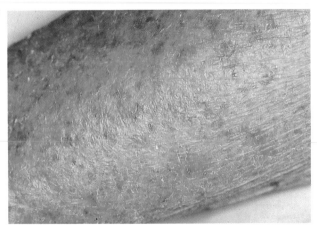

67 This condition of the skin is a frequent finding in the elderly.
(a) What is it called?
(b) What are the congenital forms of this disorder in the elderly?
(c) What are the acquired forms?

68 (a) What abnormalities are seen in this blood film?
(b) What are the clinical features of this condition in the elderly?

68

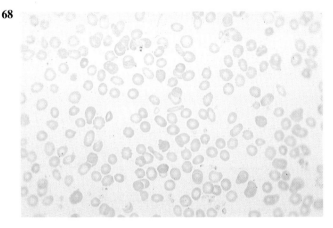

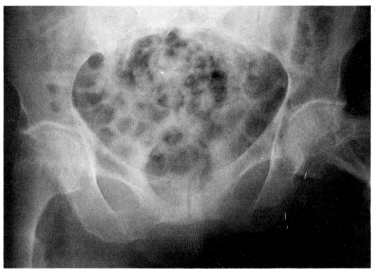

69 This elderly patient presented with urinary incontinence.
(a) What underlying problem is suggested by the X-ray of the pelvis?
(b) How should this case be treated?

70 (a) What abnormality is shown in this X-ray
of the skull?
(b) Describe the bone pathology.
(c) List the different clinical features.

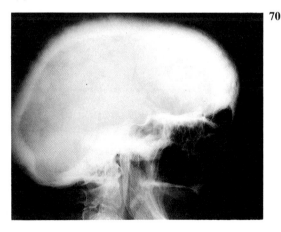

71

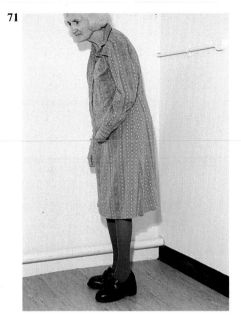

71 (a) What condition is suggested by the posture of this patient?
(b) What is the basic neurological defect in this disorder?
(c) What is the prognosis in the elderly?

72

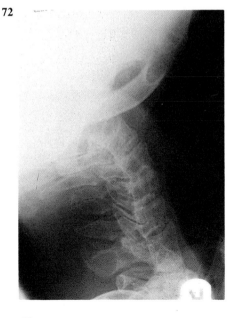

72 (a) What diagnosis is suggested by this X-ray of the cervical spine?
(b) What are the associated clinical features in the elderly?

73 (a) What is the bony abnormality?
(b) How is pain controlled in this condition?

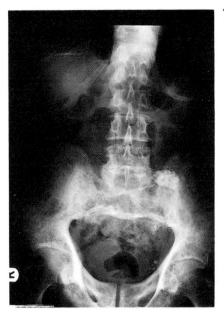

74 (a) What is this condition due to?
(b) What clinical features are seen in face and head?

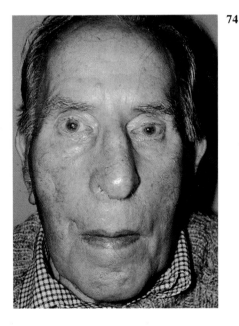

75 (a) What is this condition?
(b) What are the common findings in the mouths of otherwise healthy old people?

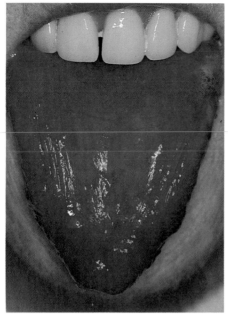

76 (a) What is this patient being treated for?
(b) What is the most likely underlying problem?
(c) What is the long-term complication if this condition is inadequately treated?

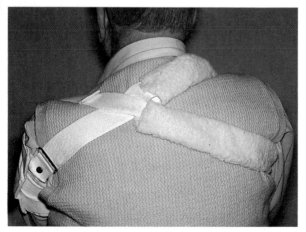

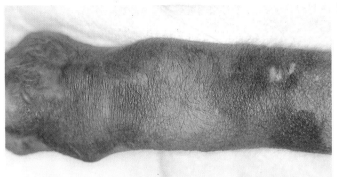

77 This elderly patient has been on long-term steroids for asthma.
(a) What is this abnormality?
(b) What other skin changes may be present?
(c) Name other neuromuscular complications of long-term glucocorticoid therapy?

78 This 85 year old patient presented with acute arthritis of the knee joint.
(a) What abnormality is shown in the X-ray?
(b) How can you confirm the diagnosis?

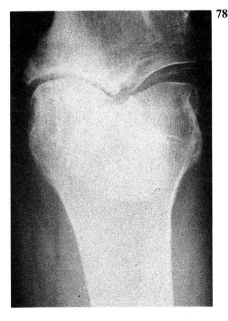

79

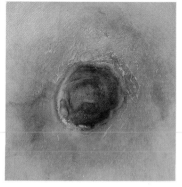
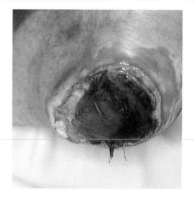
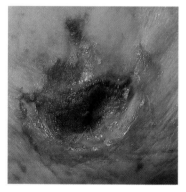

79 (a) What are the main predisposing factors that lead to pressure sores?
(b) What are the principals of treatment?

80 This elderly man was admitted as an emergency with acute confusion. He was unkempt and yellowish stains were noted on his clothing and hands.
(a) What is the underlying problem?
(b) How should he be managed?

80

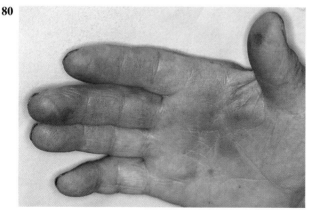

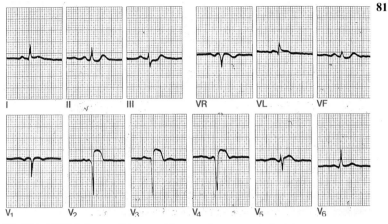

81 This ECG is from a 76 year old man who presented with acute agitation and disorientation.
(a) What does the ECG show?
(b) What are the common manifestations of this condition in elderly patients?

82 (a) What is the diagnosis?
(b) What are the likely causes of this condition?

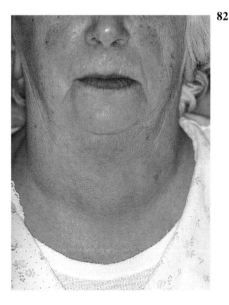

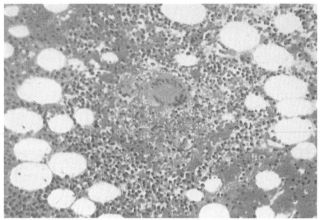

83 (a) What diagnosis is suggested by this histological picture of the bone marrow?
(b) How does this condition present in the elderly?

84 (a) What does this X-ray show?
(b) What are the symptoms?
(c) What are the causes of painful and stiff shoulder in the elderly?

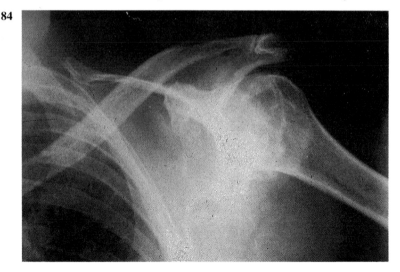

85 (a) What are the pathological features of this condition?
(b) What are the criteria for suspecting malignant change in pigmented skin lesions?

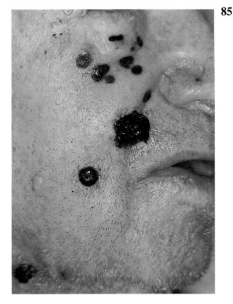

86 (a) What does this plain X-ray of the abdomen show?
(b) What are the common causes of this condition in the elderly?

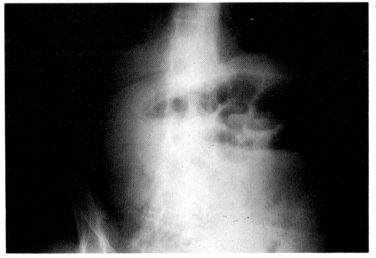

87

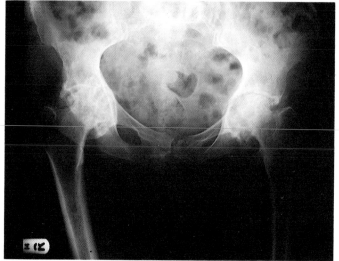

87 (a) Describe this X-ray.
(b) What are the principles of treatment?

88 This elderly patient has painless hepatomegaly.
(a) How would you investigate this case?
(b) What are the likely causes?

88

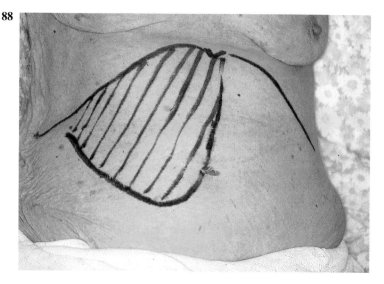

89 This is a common condition in elderly female patients.
(a) What is it?
(b) What problems does it cause in the elderly?

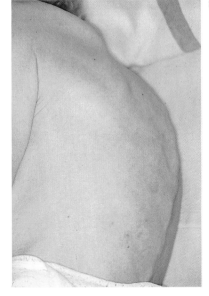

90 (a) Describe this condition.
(b) What is the most frequent presenting complaint?
(c) What is the basic pathological abnormality?

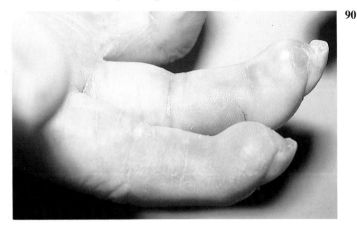

91

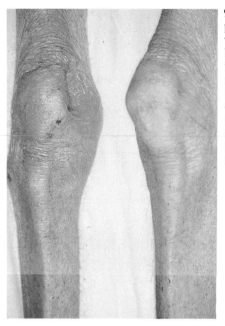

91 This elderly man has progressive wasting and weakness of limbs with hyper-reflexia in the legs and fasciculations in the arm muscles.
(a) What is the likely diagnosis?
(b) What are the different types of this condition?
(c) What is the differential diagnosis?

92 This patient has generalized pruritus.
(a) What are its common systemic causes in the elderly?
(b) What are the causes of severe pruritus due to skin disease?

92

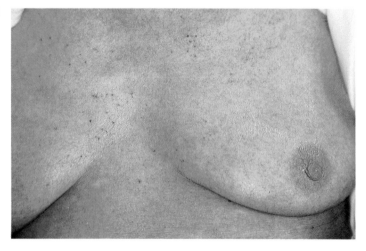

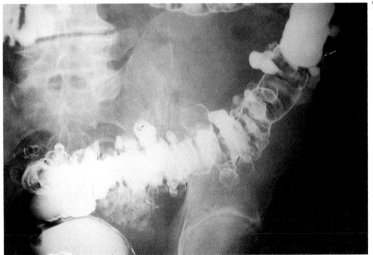

93 (a) What does this X-ray show?
(b) What are the common symptoms in this condition?
(c) What complications may occur?

94 (a) What is this condition?
(b) What is the treatment?

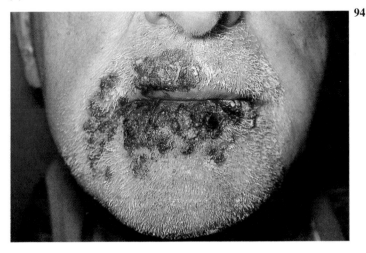

95 (a) What does this X-ray show?
(b) What is the aetiology of this condition in the elderly?
(c) What are the different types of fractures of the neck of the femur?

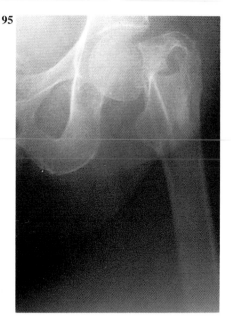

96 (a) What does this X-ray show?
(b) Which tests may help in determining the nature of a euthyroid goitre?

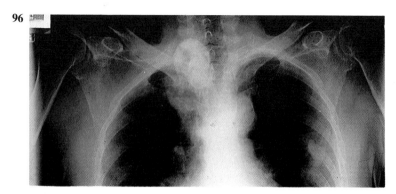

97 (a) What does this X-ray show?
(b) What symptoms will the patient have?
(c) Which is the single most important investigation in this case?

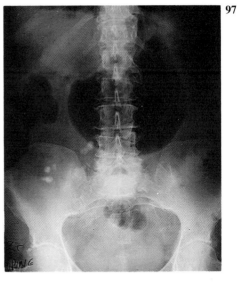

98 (a) What is this condition called?
(b) How does this develop in the elderly?

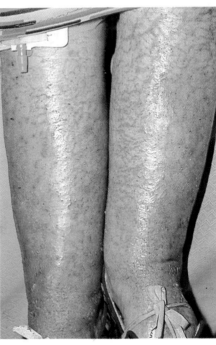

99

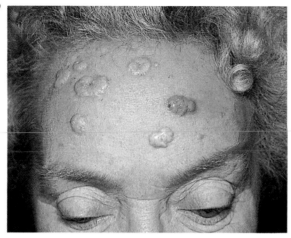

99 (a) What is this condition?
(b) What other skin condition looks very similar?

100 (a) This X-ray shows a common condition in the elderly. What is it?
(b) What are the clinical features?

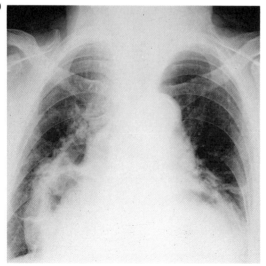

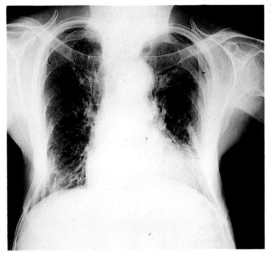

101 (a) What is unusual about the shape of this thorax?
(b) What further investigations are needed?

102 (a) What is the significance of this radiological sign?
(b) What conditions may this be confused with?

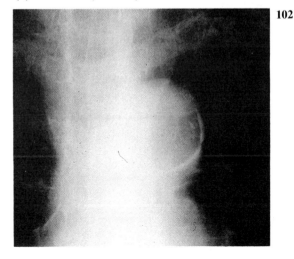

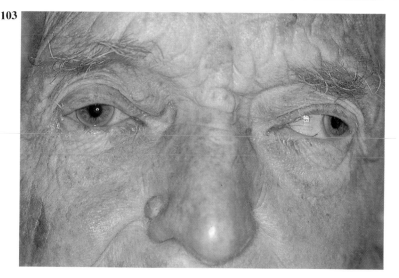

103 This elderly man complained of diplopia.
(a) Where is the lesion?
(b) What may be the underlying causes?

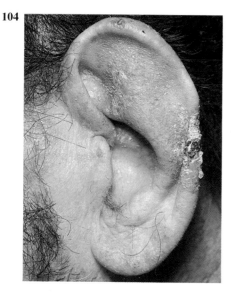

104 (a) What is the lesion on the ear?
(b) What are the predisposing factors?
(c) What treatment is recommended?

105 This patient has chronic obstructive airways disease.
(a) What does the picture show?
(b) What abnormalities do you expect to see in the lung function tests?

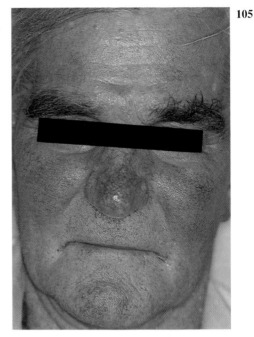

106 This endoscopic picture is from a patient who was complaining of dyspepsia and heartburn.
(a) What does it show?
(b) What is the treatment?

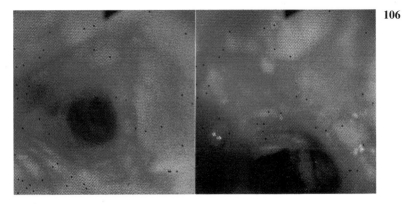

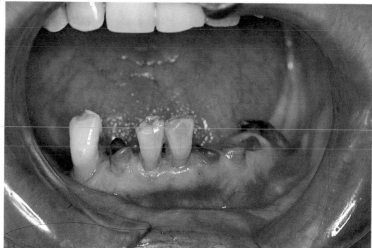

107 (a) What are the two most common causes of loss of teeth with advancing age?
(b) What are the risks to the patient?

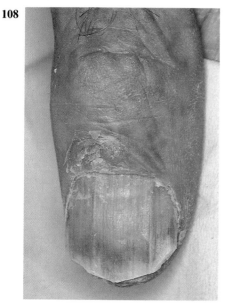

108 (a) What is wrong with this nail?
(b) Give two common causes of this appearance.

58

109 (a) What is this condition?
(b) What is its aetiology in the elderly?

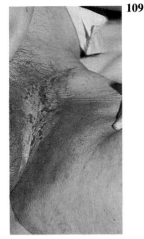

110 This patient presented with malaise, backache and weight loss, and was found to have microscopic haematuria.
(a) What does the chest X-ray show?
(b) What is the likely diagnosis?
(c) What other clinical features may be present?

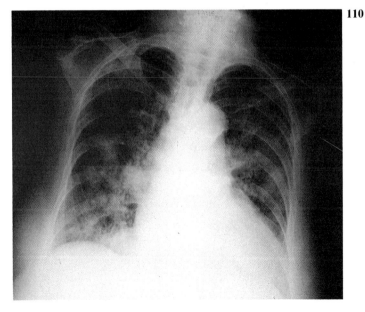

111

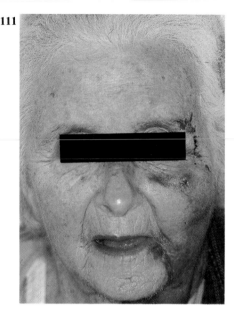

111 This 86 year old woman presented with recurrent falls resulting in facial injuries.
(a) What are the general features of falls in the elderly?
(b) What are the common complications of such falls?

112 This patient was admitted with dehydration and abdominal discomfort.
(a) What is the most important aspect of clinical assessment?
(b) What does the pelvis X-ray show?
(c) What are the causes of this condition in the elderly?

112

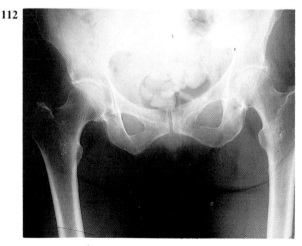

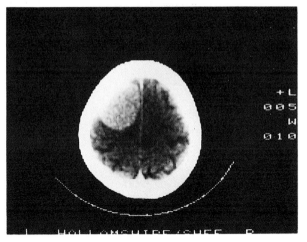

113 (a) What does this CT scan show?
(b) This lesion is involving the frontal lobe. What will the clinical features be?

114 (a) Give three common causes of this deformity of the hand.
(b) How can this problem be managed in cases of hemiplegia?

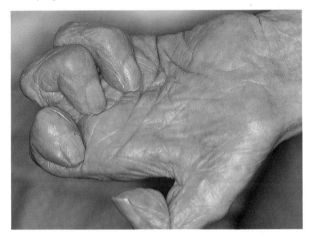

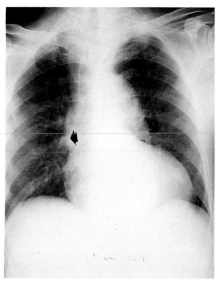

115 This elderly man presented with features of aortic regurgitation.
(a) What does the chest X-ray show?
(b) What are the causes of aortic regurgitation?

116 This elderly patient had longstanding rheumatoid arthritis and chronic dyspnoea.
(a) What does the chest X-ray show?
(b) What are the pulmonary complications associated with rheumatoid disease?

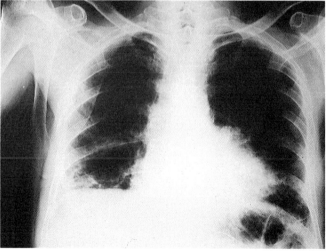

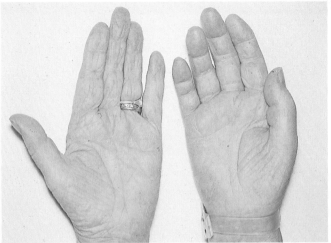

117 This patient has right-sided hemiplegia.
(a) What does the picture show?
(b) How would you manage this case?

118 (a) What does this bone marrow show?
(b) How does the renal damage occur in this condition?

118

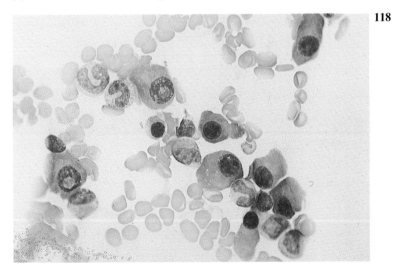

119

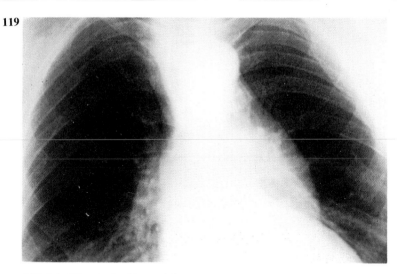

119 (a) What is the diagnosis?
(b) What is the aetiology of this condition?

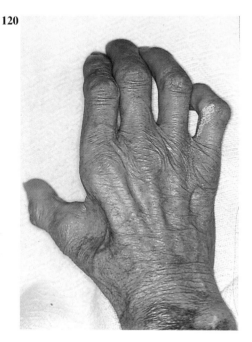

120 (a) What is the main abnormality in this hand?
(b) What are the likely causes in elderly patients?

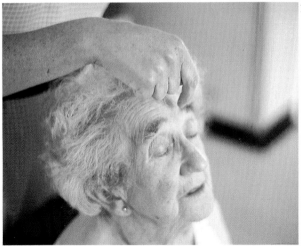

121 (a) What sign is being demonstrated?
(b) In which condition is this sign positive?

122 (a) What abnormality is shown in this X-ray?
(b) What further investigations are required?

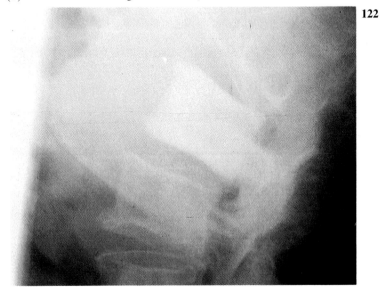

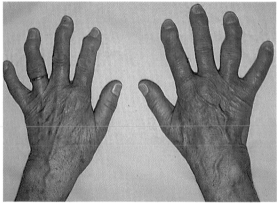

123 (a) What classical sign is shown in these hands?
(b) What is the underlying condition?
(c) What are its early symptoms?

124 This chest X-ray belongs to an acutely ill 90 year old.
(a) What is the diagnosis?
(b) What are the clinical features of this condition in elderly patients?

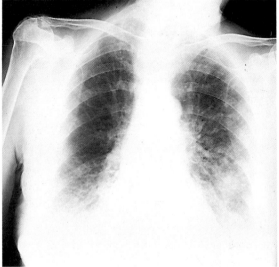

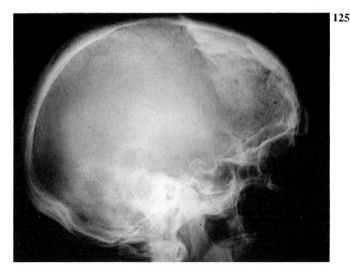

125 (a) What is this abnormality?
(b) What are the clinical features?
(c) What is the differential diagnosis?

126 (a) What abnormalities are seen in this specimen?
(b) What clinical features accompany these abnormalities in the elderly?

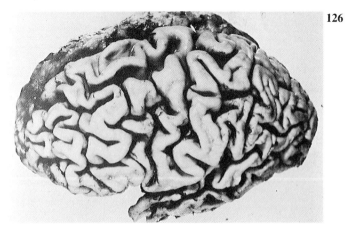

127

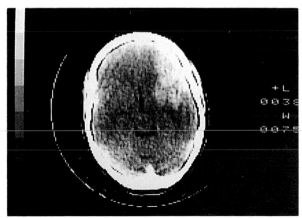

127 This CT scan shows recent middle cerebral artery infarct.
(a) What are the main clinical features of this condition?
(b) In stroke illness, which features indicate a poor prognosis?

128 (a) What is this skin condition?
(b) What does it indicate?
(c) What are the skin markers of internal malignant disease?

128

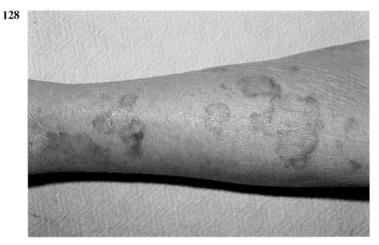

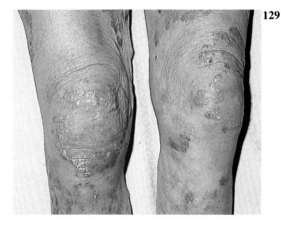

129 (a) What is this condition?
(b) What factors in the history may help in
making a diagnosis?
(c) What are the main types of this condition?

130 (a) What are these
lesions?
(b) What are the causes of
secondary osteoarthritis?

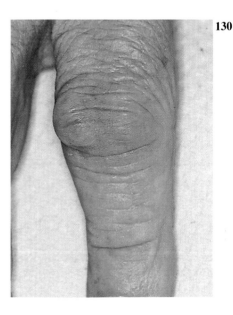

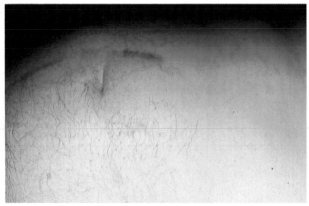

131 (a) What is this sign called?
(b) What is it due to?
(c) At which sites in the body might you find this abnormality?

132 This patient has fungating carcinoma of the breast.
(a) What is the incidence of CA breast?
(b) What investigations should be done after clinical assessment?

133 This elderly female
patient complains of severe
backache.
(a) What does the X-ray
show?
(b) What is the aetiology of
this bone disorder?

133

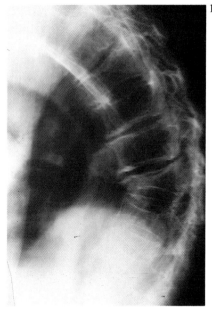

134 These neurofibrillary tangles come from a case of senile
dementia.
(a) What are they composed of?
(b) What are the different types of chronic non-organic
dementias?

134

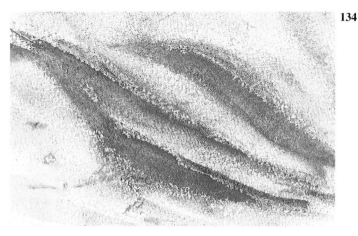

135

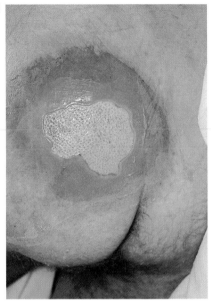

135 This elderly patient fell in the kitchen.
(a) What are the likely causes of this lesion?
(b) What are the cardiovascular causes of falls in the elderly?

136 (a) What does this picture of bone histology show?
(b) What are the clinical features of this condition?

136

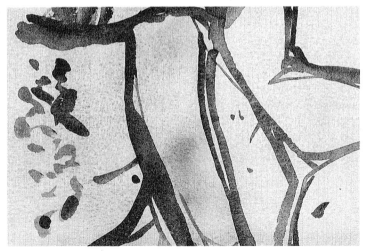

137 (a) What are the complications of this condition?
(b) What is the treatment?

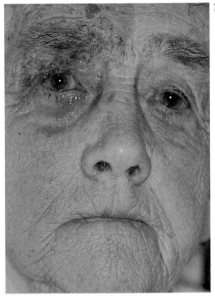

138 (a) Describe the pathology of this specimen?
(b) How did the patient present?

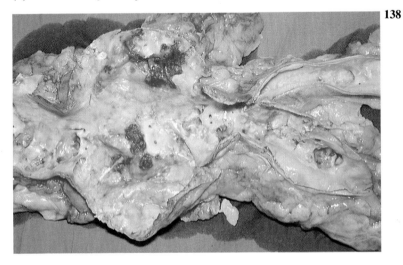

139

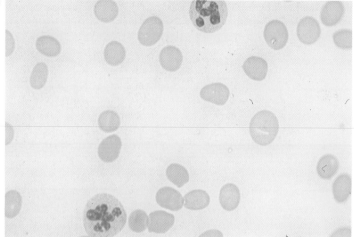

139 (a) What does this picture show?
(b) What are the causes of this condition?
(c) What are the clinical features?

140 (a) What is this fundal appearance typical of?
(b) What are the causes of sudden blindness in the elderly?

140

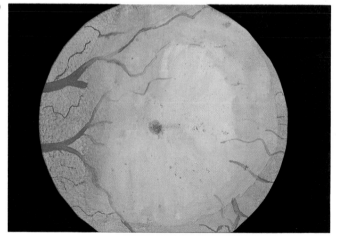

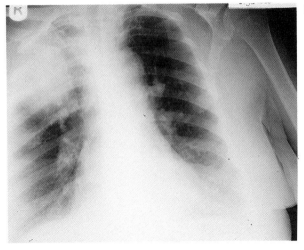

141 (a) What is the diagnosis?
(b) What are the endocrine syndromes associated with this condition?

142 (a) What is this abnormality?
(b) What are the causes?
(c) What are the features of Horner's syndrome?

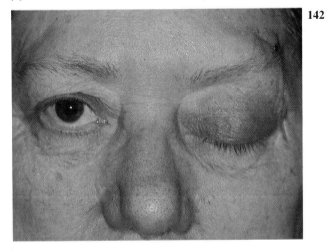

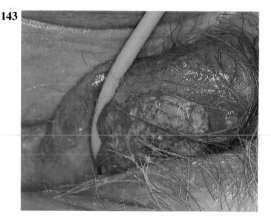

143 This patient presented with urinary incontinence.
(a) What is the cause in this case?
(b) What abnormalities are seen in the bladders of normal elderly people who may also have urinary incontinence?
(c) What are the causes of persistent (established) urinary incontinence in the elderly?

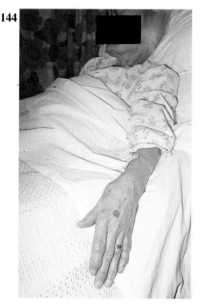

144 This elderly patient was admitted with hypothermia. Note the cyanosis.
(a) Why are elderly people so vulnerable to hypothermia?
(b) What are the main complications of hypothermia?

145 This picture is from a case of pemphigus.
(a) What sign is being demonstrated?
(b) What are the typical histological features of pemphigus?
(c) Give four causes of bullous skin lesions in the elderly.

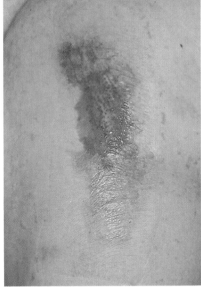

145

146 (a) What does this ECG show?
(b) What are the causes of this arrhythmia in the elderly?

146

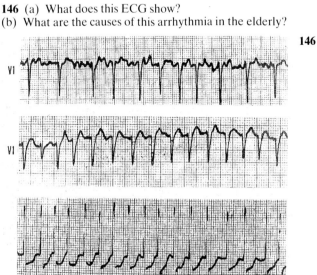

147

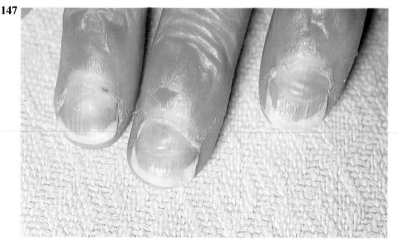

147 (a) What signs are present in these nails?
(b) What are the features of arthritis associated with this condition?

148 Wasting of some of the small muscles of the hand.
(a) Which nerve is involved?
(b) Which muscles does it innervate?
(c) How would you confirm the diagnosis?

148

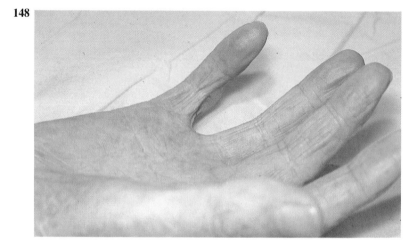

149 (a) What is the diagnosis?
(b) What are the cutaneous features of this condition?
(c) What are the special features of this disorder in the elderly?

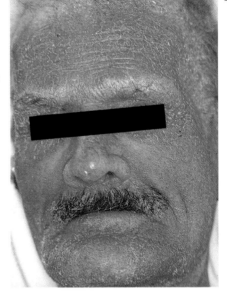

149

150 (a) What does this CT scan show?
(b) What is the clinical diagnosis?
(c) What are the clinical features in the elderly?

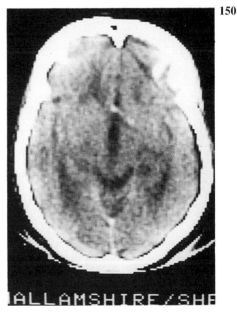

150

151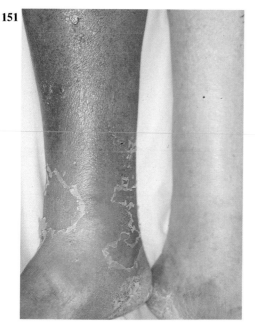

151 (a) What is this condition?
(b) What should it be distinguished from?
(c) What is the treatment?

152 This patient presented acutely.
(a) What does the CT scan show?
(b) What are the clinical features of this condition?

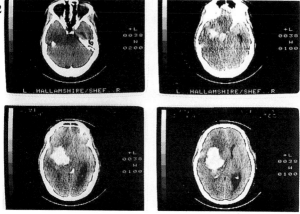

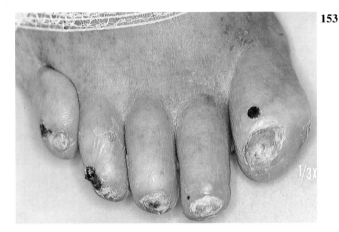

153 This patient presented with dyspnoea, pyrexia, anaemia and cardiac failure. Lesions shown in the picture were present in the toes of both feet.
(a) What is the likely diagnosis?
(b) Which is the commonest causative organism?
(c) What are the special features of this illness in the elderly?

154 (a) What is this lesion?
(b) What are the secondary causes of this condition?

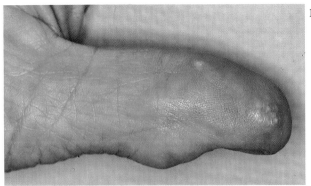

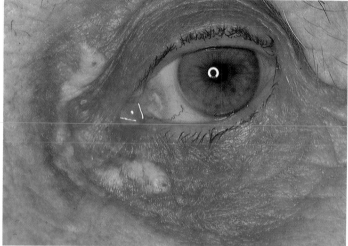

155 (a) What are these lesions?
(b) What is the most likely underlying disorder?
(c) What is the main risk to the patient?

156 (a) What does this CT scan show?
(b) What are the clinical features of such lesions?

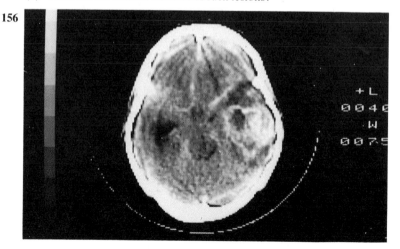

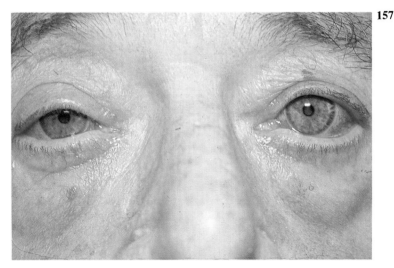

157 This patient has irritation and watering of both eyes.
(a) What is the likely diagnosis?
(b) What is the common causative agent?

158 This elderly patient has right-sided primary pneumonia.
(a) What organisms cause primary pneumonia?
(b) What are the special features of viral pneumonia?

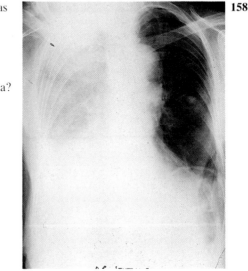

159

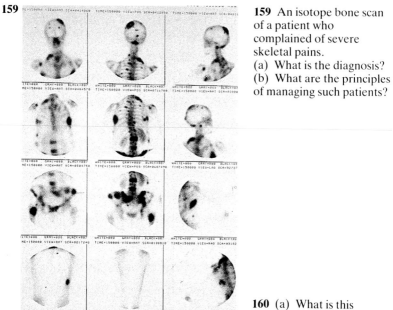

159 An isotope bone scan of a patient who complained of severe skeletal pains.
(a) What is the diagnosis?
(b) What are the principles of managing such patients?

160 (a) What is this condition?
(b) What is its aetiology?

160

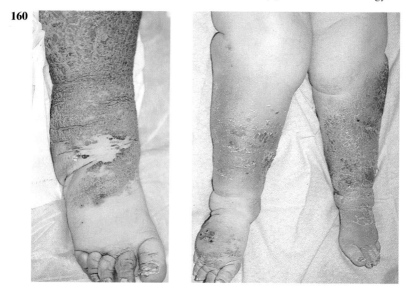

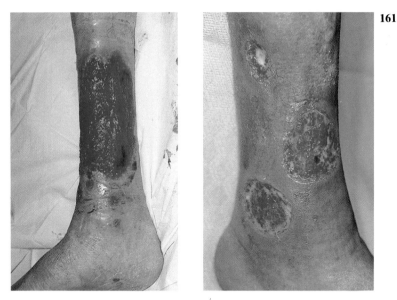

161 (a) What are the causes of leg ulcers in the elderly?
(b) What are the features of arterial leg ulcers?

162 (a) What is the obvious abnormality?
(b) What are the causes of this condition secondary to ocular disease?

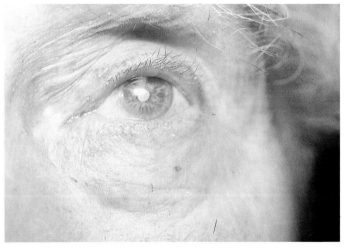

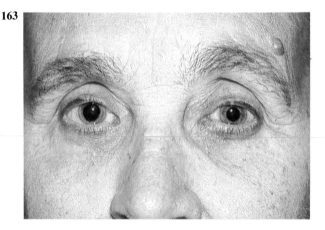

163 (a) What is the ocular abnormality?
(b) What are the likely causes?

164 (a) What is this abnormality?
(b) What problems can this condition cause in the elderly?

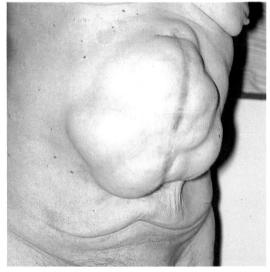

165 This patient has generalized hyperpigmentation.
(a) What are the endocrine causes of diffuse hyperpigmentation in the elderly?
(b) Give three causes of non-melanin pigmentation.

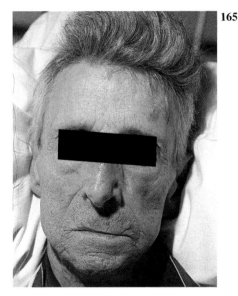

165

166 (a) What is the cause of this intense itching of the leg?
(b) What is its distribution on the body?
(c) What chemicals are used in treatment?

166

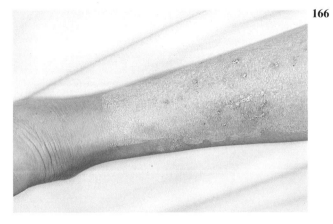

167

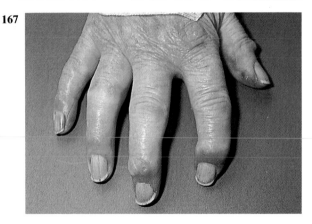

167 (a) What is the diagnosis?
(b) Describe this condition.
(c) Give ten causes.

168 This patient is a case of Parkinsonism who came into hospital with an acute problem.
(a) What is the likely diagnosis?
(b) In what types of Parkinsonism does this problem occur?

168

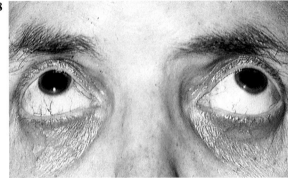

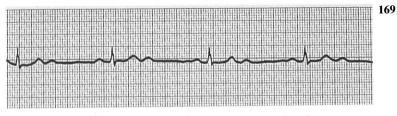

169 (a) What biochemical abnormality does this ECG show?
(b) Give five clinical features that occur due to this biochemical abnormality.

170 (a) Which type of leukaemia is seen in this blood film?
(b) What changes occur in the bone marrow?

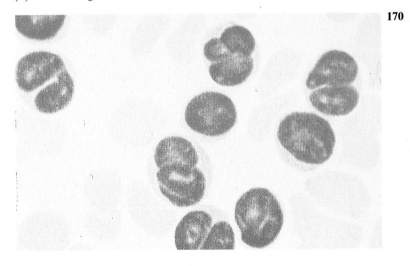

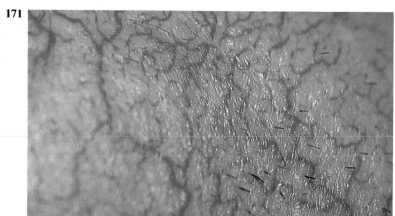

171 The cheek of an elderly farmer.
(a) What are these changes?
(b) What are they due to?

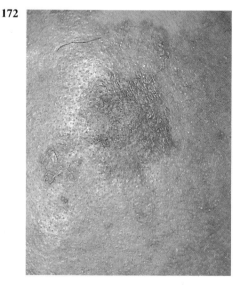

172 (a) What is this non-symptomatic lesion in an elderly man?
(b) What is it due to?
(c) Give two differential diagnoses.

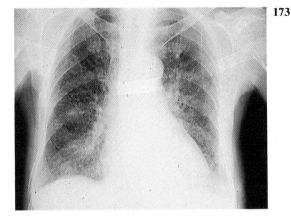

173 This man, who was a retired industrial worker, complained of increasing dyspnoea of some years' duration.
(a) What diagnosis is suggested by the chest X-ray?
(b) What defects may be present in the lung function tests?
(c) Which inorganic substances cause this problem?

174 This woman presented with haematuria and renal failure.
(a) Name two abnormalities seen in the X-ray.
(b) Give five causes of dark-coloured urine.

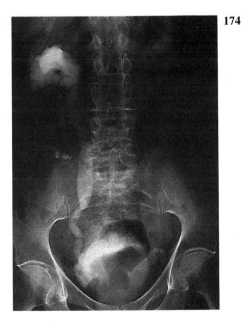

175

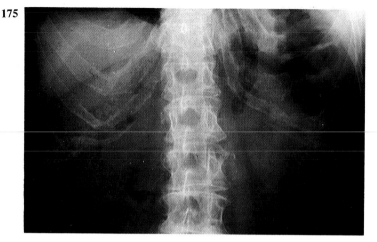

175 (a) What does this X-ray show?
(b) What is the pathological significance of this finding in elderly patients?

176 This patient was admitted as an emergency with a history of deep vein thrombosis.
(a) What does the lung scan show?
(b) Which clinical features may accompany this pathology?

176

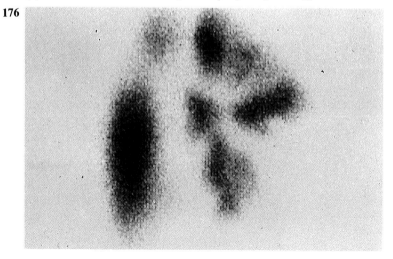

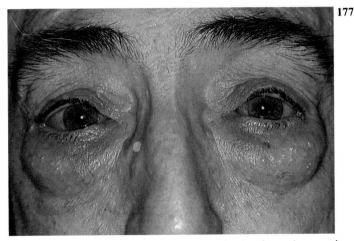

177 This patient presented with a history of polyuria, oedema and anaemia.
(a) What abnormality is seen in the face?
(b) What is the likely diagnosis?
(c) Give three conditions that can cause similar facial appearance.

178 This elderly female patient presented with gross distension of the abdomen of long standing.
(a) Give five causes of such abdominal distension.
(b) What are the main types of primary ovarian tumours?
(c) What are the complications of ovarian cyst?

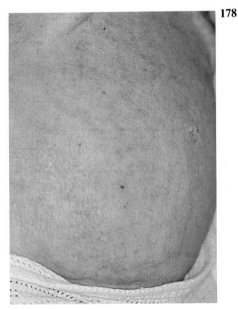

179

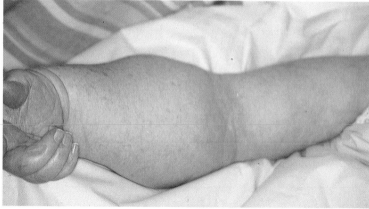

179 (a) What abnormality is seen in this arm?
(b) What is the most likely underlying pathology?
(c) Name three newer methods of detecting the primary pathology.

180 (a) Name the lesion seen on the back of the hand of this elderly man.
(b) What is the aetiology?

180

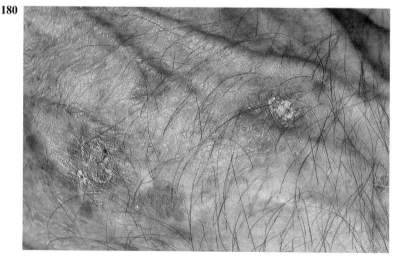

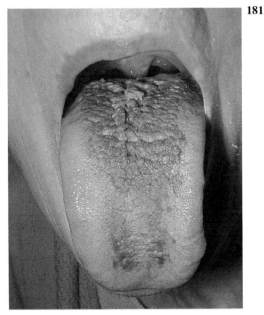

181 (a) What are the causes of dark discoloration of the tongue?
(b) Why is this appearance sometimes called 'black-hairy tongue'?

182 This ECG shows features of sick sinus syndrome.
(a) Describe the syndrome.
(b) Which symptoms occur with this condition?

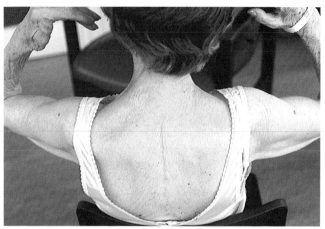

183 This patient presented with 'rheumatism', especially around the shoulders and pelvis, plus anaemia. She is unable to lift her arms above shoulder level.
(a) What is the likely diagnosis?
(b) Which investigations will confirm the diagnosis?
(c) What is the natural history of this condition?

184 Hypertensive fundus from an elderly patient with poorly controlled hypertension.
(a) What are the main features in this fundus?
(b) What is the incidence of strokes in hypertensive patients?
(c) What are the general guidelines for treating hypertension in the elderly?

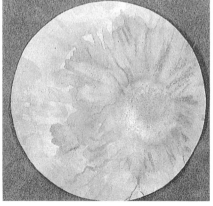

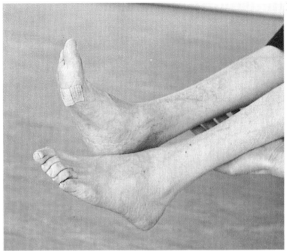

185 This patient has developed a left foot drop following a stroke.
(a) Which nerve is involved?
(b) What is the most common cause of foot drop in cases of hemiplegia?

186 This patient has developed looseness of dentures following a stroke.
(a) What is the cause?
(b) What further complications may occur?

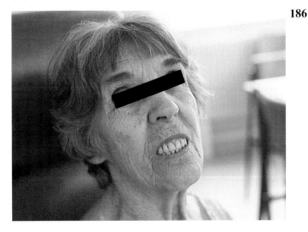

187

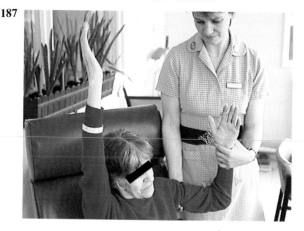

187 This elderly patient has developed a painful 'frozen shoulder'.
(a) What is a 'frozen shoulder'?
(b) What are the typical radiological features?

188 This hearing aid belongs to an elderly patient who was using it incorrectly.
(a) What are the problems associated with untreated deafness in the elderly?
(b) What are the common causes of deafness in the elderly?

188

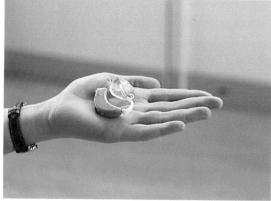

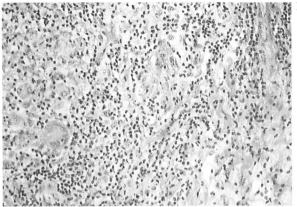

189 Histological picture of temporal artery biopsy.
(a) What does this show?
(b) What are the clinical features associated with this condition?

190 This is a picture of the fundus of an elderly man who was complaining of deteriorating vision over a number of years.
(a) What is the most likely cause of his deteriorating vision?
(b) What is the classical sign of this condition?

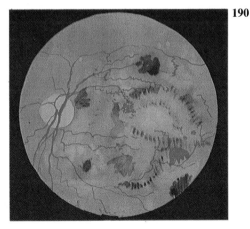

190

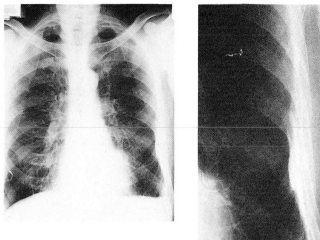

191 (a) What abnormality is seen in this chest X-ray?
(b) What are the different types of asbestos-related diseases of the lungs and pleura?

192 This patient has an indwelling catheter for the management of transient urinary incontinence.
(a) What are the main types of transient (reversible) urinary incontinence?
(b) What are the disadvantages of long-term catheterization?

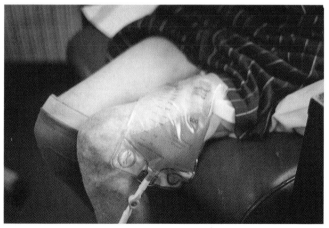

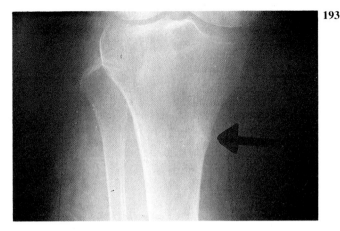

193 This 88 year old presented with rheumatic aches and pains and immobility.
(a) What does the X-ray show?
(b) What is the diagnosis?
(c) What is the underlying condition due to?

194 This patient presented with myocardial infarction leading to severe cardiac failure, hypoxia and uraemia. Within a few hours he developed extensive purpura and ecchymosis.
(a) What is the most likely diagnosis?
(b) Which other conditions can cause this complication?

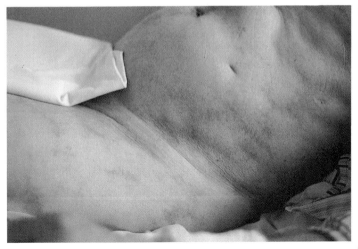

195

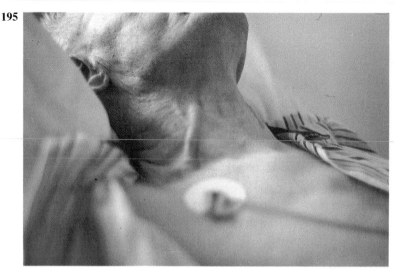

195 This patient has elevated jugular venous pressure.
(a) What is the most important cause of raised jugular venous pressure?
(b) Name two other causes of raised JVP in the elderly.

196

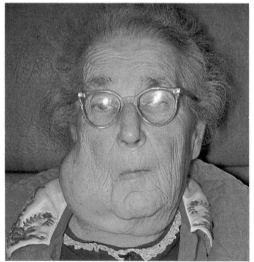

196 (a) Which tissue is involved in this facial swelling?
(b) Give three causes.

197 (a) Describe this condition of the skin.
(b) Which auto-immune disorders are associated with this sign?

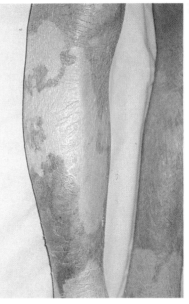

197

198 This condition of the scalp is seen frequently in the elderly.
(a) What is it?
(b) Name five other conditions which can give rise to a similar clinical picture.

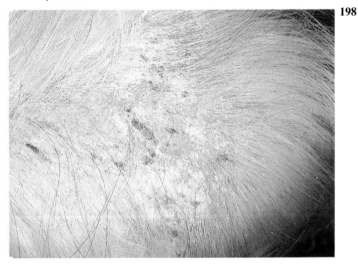

198

199

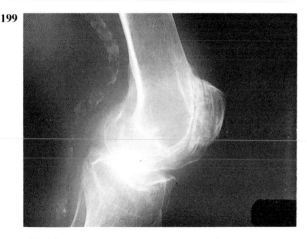

199 (a) Name two abnormalities seen in this X-ray.
(b) Are these two conditions linked?

200 (a) What is this abnormality of the hand?
(b) Which method is used by the occupational therapists in treating and rehabilitating stroke patients?

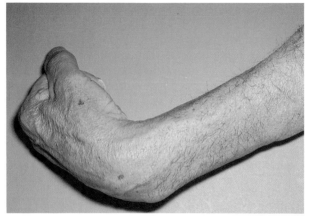

ANSWERS

1 (a) Deep vein thrombosis and infection in the right knee prosthesis.
(b) Pulmonary embolism and septicaemia. She is also at risk from all the complications of being bedfast, ie pressure sores, incontinence, depression, loss of mobility and pneumonia.

2 (a) The patient has purpura. In the elderly, the likely causes are senile purpura, steroid induced purpura, uraemia, hypothermia and idiopathic or secondary thrombocytopenic purpura.
(b) Haemoglobin estimation, platelet count, plasma viscosity, urea and electrolytes, clotting screen, leucocyte ascorbic acid level, and if necessary bone marrow examination.

3 (a) Glossitis caused by Candida infection.
(b) Poor oral hygiene, frequent use of antibiotics, dentures, stomatitis, severe and prolonged debilitating states and leukaemias.

4 (a) Rehabilitation is best carried out in a specialist geriatric rehabilitation ward with a multidisciplinary approach. Therapists and a clinical psychologist should be available. There should be access to an Artificial Limb and Appliance Centre. Relatives should be involved in rehabilitation.
(b) Problems after limb amputation include phantom limb sensations and pains, grief reactions, depression, psychosocial problems, loss of occupation and negative attitudes to the prosthesis.

5 (a) Haemorrhoids.
(b) Severe pain increasing with defaecation, constipation, faecal impaction, faecal incontinence, blood loss leading to anaemia or even shock.

6 (a) Cushing's syndrome.
(b) The cause of Cushing's syndrome can be divided into two groups: (1) *ACTH-dependent causes*—iatrogenic, Cushing's disease, ectopic ACTH syndrome; (2) *non-ACTH-dependent causes*—iatrogenic, adenomas or carcinoma of the adrenal cortex.

7 (a) Erythema multiforme.
(b) Bullous erythema multiforme with high fever, oral bullae and stomatitis, conjunctivitis, uveitis, corneal ulcers, urethritis, balanitis, vulvo-vaginitis, chest infection and polyarthritis.

8 (a) Calcification of the abdominal aorta and splenic artery.
(b) No. Calcification of the abdominal aorta is a common finding in the elderly, and is due to widespread aortic atheroma. Sometimes it is associated with aneurysmal dilatation of the aorta which may subsequently leak or rupture. It may be confused with other causes of abdominal calcification, eg pancreatic calcification, calcified fibroid, calcified lymph nodes, phleboliths, faecaliths.

9 (a) Haemoglobin, ESR or plasma viscosity, plasma urea, plasma proteins and protein electrophoresis, Bence-Jones proteins in the urine, serum calcium, radiological survey of the skeleton and bone marrow examination.
(b) Bone pains, pathological fractures, peripheral neuropathy, anaemia, renal failure and nephrotic syndrome, recurrent infections, hyperviscosity syndrome, bleeding and amyloidosis.

10 (a) Angular stomatitis.
(b) This patient should be investigated for anaemia and vitamin deficiency. Check haemoglobin, serum ferritin, red cell folate and serum vitamin B12. Poor oral hygiene, chronic gum disease and ill-fitting dentures may also contribute to this condition.

11 (a) The X-ray shows features suggestive of mitral stenosis. Typical auscultatory findings are loud tapping apex beat and opening snap, characteristic diastolic murmur often with a thrill. Accompanying mitral regurgitation may cause a pansystolic murmur. Pulmonary hypertension causes a loud pulmonary component of the second heart sound.
(b) Complications include cardiac failure, atrial fibrillation, pulmonary hypertension, cerebral embolism and sometimes pulmonary tuberculosis.

12 (a) The main abnormalities are wasting of the small muscles, ulnar deviation of the fingers and hand, and swelling and deformity of all proximal interphalangeal joints.
(b) This is a case of chronic severe, probably burnt-out rheumatoid arthritis. In the elderly it is less common in males, and systemic features such as weight loss, lymphadenopathy, splenomegaly and prolonged morning stiffness are of less intensity. The onset tends to be abrupt and anaemia and high ESR are both common. Nodules are less frequent but osteoporosis appears early. Also arteritis is rare in older patients.

13 (a) Chloramphenicol, anti-tuberculous drugs, phenacetin and alcohol.
(b) Primary sideroblastic anaemia is inherited and may respond to pyridoxine. The secondary variety occurs in association with myeloproliferative disorders, collagen diseases, myxoedema, cutaneous porphyria and lead poisoning. The diagnostic feature is hypochromic anaemia with 'ring sideroblasts' in the bone marrow—as illustrated.

14 (a) The patient is probably living in a state of neglect and deprivation in a house which is cold. She has been sitting too near the fire to keep warm.
(b) The patient should be investigated for anaemia, malnutrition and hypothyroidism. She will also require a thorough domiciliary assessment, preferably by an occupational therapist and a social worker.

15 (a) Dupuytren's contracture.
(b) There is a high incidence in patients with liver disease, chronic alcoholism and epilepsy.
(c) Selective fasciectomy.

16 (a) The CT scan shows right hemisphere space occupying lesion, probably glioma. Clinical features are: (1) *general symptoms*—headache, confusion, behaviour disorders, epilepsy and dementia; (2) *localizing features*—hemiparesis, hemianopia, diplopia, cranial nerve palsies; (3) *false localizing signs*—secondary to raised intracranial pressure, 6th nerve palsy, cerebellar ataxia.
(b) The patient requires a detailed neurosurgical evaluation. Surgery in the elderly is usually not possible. However some patients may benefit from palliative surgery—partial removal or drainage of the cyst, decompression and relief of intracranial pressure. A short-circuiting procedure may relieve internal hydrocephalus. Radiotherapy is sometimes useful in relieving symptoms. Dexamethasone will reduce the elevated intracranial pressure and relieve symptoms such as headache, drowsiness, nausea and vomiting.

17 (a) Venous insufficiency, gravitational factors plus immobility, cardiac failure, hypoproteinaemia, lymphoedema and hepatic failure.
(b) Urinary incontinence, skin rashes, nausea and vomiting, hypo- and hyperkalaemia, gout, glucose intolerance and postural hypotension.

18 (a) Hereditary haemorrhagic telangiectasia.
(b) Epistaxis, haematemesis, haemoptysis and anaemia.

19 (a) Sore on the plantar surface of the foot giving rise to pain and instability. The sore is due to diabetes mellitus plus ill-fitting footwear.
(b) Tripping over objects, slipping, wearing old and ill-fitting footwear, slippery surfaces, narrow steep stairs, poor lighting, pets, electrical flexes, rolled up edges of carpets and mats. Falls are also common during physiotherapy and rehabilitation, especially in patients recovering from strokes.

20 (a) Symptoms of gall stones and OA spine: nausea, anorexia, right hypochondrial pain, weight loss and jaundice; also backache, pain radiating down the legs and immobility.
(b) Cholesterol gall stones are most common (up to 75%). The remaining 25% of the stones are calcium bilirubinate (pigment stones) which are either black or brown in colour.

21 (a) Recent right middle cerebral artery infarct.
(b) Hemiparesis, hemianopia, cortical sensory loss, disturbance of attention, loss of recognition of body image plus other perceptual problems.

22 (a) The picture shows calcification at the corneoscleral junction. Other features of hypercalcaemia include weakness, anorexia, nausea, vomiting, constipation, drowsiness or confusion. Less frequent complications include peptic ulceration, acute pancreatitis, pseudo-gout and hypertension.
(b) The causes of hypercalcaemia are hyperparathyroidism, bony metastases, carcinomas producing parathyroid hormone-like substances, sarcoidosis, overdosage with vitamin D, Paget's disease of the bone and chronic immobility.

23 (a) Claw-hand deformity and wasting of the small muscles of the hand due to ulnar nerve palsy.
(b) Ulnar nerve palsy may be due to trauma, compression at the elbow and diabetes mellitus. Other causes are cervical spondylosis, lesions in the cord, cervical rib, Pancoast's tumour, scalenus anterior syndrome and polyneuropathy.

24 (a) Cardiac amyloidosis. The amyloid is stained green, muscle yellow and fibrous tissue red.
(b) Increasing congestive cardiac failure of obscure origin.

25 (a) Inadequate clinical assessment, excessive prescribing, inadequate supervision of long-term medication, altered pharmacokinetics and pharmacodynamics in the elderly and poor compliance.
(b) Compliance can be improved by making the drug regime simpler to understand and the medication physically easier to take. Measures may also include patient instruction and counselling, clearly written instructions, transparent glass or plastic containers with wing-nut lids, clearer labelling, memory aids such as calendar packs and Dosett boxes, long-term supervision, and guidance from the ward or surgery pharmacists.

26 (a) Hypothyroidism.
(b) Neuropathy, hypothermia, falls and immobility, myxoedema coma, dementia, carpal tunnel syndrome, pericardial effusion, ascites and cerebellar ataxia.
(c) Thyroxine. Start with small doses (25 mcg or 50 mcg daily), especially if there is evidence of ischaemic heart disease. After two to three weeks the dose can be increased by 50 mcg. The usual maintenance dose is between 100 and 200 mcg daily. The effectiveness of hormone replacement is assessed by clinical improvement and measuring TSH levels. The patient's follow up should be for life.

27 (a) Torticollis.
(b) Diseases of the extrapyramidal system, especially Parkinsonism, chorea, ballism and athetosis. It is a frequent complication in patients with schizophrenia who are on long-term Phenothiazine drugs.

28 (a) Candidosis (moniliasis) due to infection by *Candida albicans*.
(b) Mild superficial infections respond to Nystatin. In severe cases Ketoconazole or Amphotericin should be used. Fluconazole is now available for treatment of oral and vaginal candidosis.
(c) Diabetes mellitus, urinary incontinence, anaemias, lymphomas and reticulosis.

29 (a) Section of bone showing features of advanced osteomalacia. There are wide uncalcified seams of osteoid tissue with decrease in the staining intensity of calcification fronts.
(b) General deterioration of health, anorexia, weakness, non-specific aches and pains, bone pain leading to bone tenderness, proximal myopathy giving rise to waddling gait, increased incidence of fractures, depression, skeletal deformities and eventual complete immobility.
(c) Pseudo-fractures (Looser's zones) in the cortex of bone are diagnostic.

30 (a) Erosion of the iliac bone.
(b) Increase in plasma alkaline phosphatase and hypercalcaemia.

31 (a) Olecranon bursitis causing swelling and discomfort in a case of rheumatoid arthritis.
(b) Other periarticular soft tissue manifestations include nodules, usually below elbow (20%), tenosynovitis around hands or wrists (65%), synovial cysts eg Baker's cyst behind the knee, muscle wasting and ligamentous laxity leading to hypermobility and deformities, causing ulnar deviation and atlanto-axial subluxation.

32 (a) Onychogryphosis—overgrown, claw-like toe nails.
(b) Patients usually have other features of severe neglect and deprivation. They may be housebound, immobile and also demented.
(c) Hallux valgus, bunions, corns, benign oedema, hammer toes and peripheral vascular disease.

33 (a) Senile plaque from a case of senile dementia. The plaques consist of a central amyloid core surrounded by degenerating mitochondria, lysosomes and macrophages.
(b) Neurofibrillary tangles, granulovascular degeneration, and loss of neurones with reactive gliosis.

34 (a) Extensive atheroma of distal aorta and also at the origins of both internal iliac arteries.

(b) Peripheral vascular disease is asymptomatic in the early stages. Later on the patient will complain of cold feet, numbness, paraesthesiae in feet, intermittent claudication and then rest pain, ischaemic ulcers and eventually gangrene.

35 (a) The patient may have suffered a stroke giving rise to hemiplegia, dysphasia, hemianopia, confusion and incontinence. Patients with lower motor neurone facial paralysis may have signs of other disorders that give rise to this condition, eg herpes zoster.
(b) The main types of paralysis of facial muscles are due to: (1) lesions of the fibres of upper neurones concerned with voluntary involvement; (2) lesion of the fibres of upper motor neurones concerned with emotional movement; (3) lesion of the lower motor neurones.

36 (a) Vesiculo-bullous rash of dermatitis herpetiformis.
(b) The sites most often affected are the elbows, knees, buttocks, shoulders and scalp.
(c) Gluten enteropathy with malabsorption, tumours of gastro-intestinal tract and auto-immune disorders.

37 (a) Dyspnoea, orthopnoea, paroxysmal nocturnal dyspnoea, peripheral oedema, chest pain or tightness, palpitations, faintness, tiredness, cough, nocturia and anorexia.
(b) X-ray shows features of cardiac failure. The causes are ischaemic heart disease (48.5%), hypertension, degenerative calcific changes in mitral ring or aortic cusp, cor pulmonale, senile cardiac amyloidosis, endocarditis, calcified aortic stenosis, rheumatic heart disease, mucoid degeneration of the mitral valve, myxoedema, chronic anaemia, thyrotoxicosis, Paget's disease and beriberi.

38 (a) Serum uric acid to confirm the diagnosis of gout, ESR will be raised, white cell count to detect leucocytosis and urea and creatinine clearance to assess the renal function.
(b) Acute attacks respond rapidly to Indomethacin, colchicine, Naproxen, Fenoprofen and ACTH. Long-term treatment is with Allopurinol, especially if the patient has elevated serum uric acid, tophi or impaired renal function. Probenecid may be used as an alternative or in addition to Allopurinol in resistant cases.

39 (a) Hallux valgus. This is a common problem in the elderly. The big toe is abducted so that it lies under (or on the top) of the other toes and there is a marked prominence of the first metatarsophalangeal joint with bony enlargement of the inner side of the first metatarsal head.
(b) A bursa (bunion) has formed over the enlarged first metatarsal head. This is painful, interferes with walking and may ulcerate. Ordinary footwear may aggravate the problem further.

40 (a) The patient, who is a case of hemiplegia, is being taught to walk on a specially adapted rollator frame.
(b) Painful shoulder, hemiplegic oedema, hemiplegic arthritis, spasticity, falls, depression, hyper-extension of the knee, torticollis and postural hypotension.

41 (a) Congestive cardiac failure, venous thrombosis and incompetent venous valves, prolonged immobility and hypoalbuminaemia. Other causes are lymphoedema due to pelvic tumours, Milroy's disease, hepatic failure and nephrotic syndrome.
(b) Steroids, carbenoxolone, Indomethacin and oestrogens.

42 (a) Left-sided subdural haematoma, probably chronic.

(b) Impaired memory, confusion, headache, apathy, focal epileptic fits, dysphasia, drowsiness, incontinence and dementia.

(c) Mild hemiparesis, dilatation of the homolateral pupil, papilloedema, visual impairment. If the haematoma continues to expand, brain stem signs may appear.

43 (a) The finger nail is brittle with cracking, flattening and concavity—koilonychia.

(b) Microcytosis, hypochromia, poikilocytosis, target cells, reduced mean cell volume, normal or reduced mean corpuscular haemoglobin concentration, normal or lower than expected ESR and sometimes hypersegmentation of neutrophils.

(c) Plummer-Vinson syndrome. Iron deficiency anaemia with dysphagia due to post-cricoid web.

44 (a) Calcified fibroid.

(b) Bladder calcification, bladder stones, calcified atheromatous blood vessels, old TB lymph nodes, stones in the ureter, faecaliths and phleboliths.

45 (a) Osteoporosis.

(b) Immobility, loss of confidence, toxic confusion, pressure sores, deep vein thrombosis, incontinence, constipation, contractures and hypostatic pneumonia.

46 (a) *Streptococcus pneumoniae* and/or *H. influenzae.*

(b) FEV_1 is reduced and ratio of FEV_1 to vital capacity is also low. The residual volume is increased and PaO_2 falls below normal. In advanced cases PaO_2 falls further and there is sustained rise in $PaCO_2$. PEFR is always reduced.

47 (a) Bilateral apical calcification and small left pleural effusion.

(b) Pulmonary tuberculosis.

(c) Asbestosis, sarcoidosis and pulmonary abscess.

48 (a) Malignant gastric ulcer.

(b) No symptoms in the beginning. Later on dyspepsia, anorexia, nausea, discomfort after meals and loss of weight. After that cachexia, pallor, iron deficiency, anaemia and rarely acanthosis nigricans and malignant ascites. Metastases in the liver or scalene lymph nodes may be present.

49 (a) Diabetes mellitus with neuropathy and accelerated atherosclerosis.

(b) Patients with diabetes mellitus may have fat atrophy or hypertrophy at insulin injection sites, candidiasis and furuncles, xanthomata, necrobiosis lipoidica, granuloma annulare and ischaemic changes.

50 (a) Oestrogens, Spironolactone, Reserpine, Methyldopa, Amphetamine and Digitalis can all cause gynaecomastia.

(b) Hypothyroidism, thyrotoxicosis, acromegaly, cirrhosis of the liver, carcinoma of the bronchus, lymphoma, chronic renal failure treated with dialysis and sometimes paraplegia.

51 (a) Iridectomy for cataract.

(b) Lesions of sympathetic fibres, mid-brain lesions, Pontine haemorrhage, tabes dorsalis, multiple sclerosis, diabetes mellitus, Holmes-Adie's pupil, and drugs such as atropine and morphine.

52 (a) Cerebral atrophy.

(b) Alzheimer's-type dementia.

(c) Myxoedema, vitamin B12 and folate deficiency, cerebral tumours, alcoholism, neurosyphilis, normal pressure hydrocephalus, pellagra, hypercalcaemia, chronic renal failure, non-metastatic complications of carcinomas and certain drugs, eg barbiturates.

53 (a) 'Caput medusae', jaundice, gynaecomastia, spider telangiectasis, clubbing of fingers, purpura, hyperpigmentation and Dupuytren's contractures may all occur in cirrhosis of the liver. The illustration shows palmar erythema.
(b) Ascites, variceal bleeding, hepatic encephalopathy and renal failure.

54 (a) The X-ray shows encircling string stricture of carcinoma of the colon. Clinical features vary depending on the site. In tumours of the left colon obstruction occurs early. Tumours of the right colon present with anaemia, weight loss and alteration of bowel habit. Other features are bleeding and feeling of incomplete emptying of the bowel. Tumours may be palpated.
(b) Longstanding ulcerative colitis and familial polyposis of the colon are well-known risk factors. Dietary habits and bacterial flora of the bowel are also of aetiological significance.

55 (a) Glossitis.
(b) Glossitis is usually associated with stomatitis. Causes include aphthous ulcers, alcoholism, candidosis, herpes simplex infection, pyorrhoea, Stevens-Johnson syndrome, neutropenia and leukaemias, iron deficiency, vitamin B complex including vitamin B12 and folate deficiencies, pemphigus vulgaris, lichen planus, cytotoxic drugs, certain antibiotics, potassium supplements, leucoplakia and ill-fitting dentures.

56 (a) Rhinophyma.
(b) Rosacea.
(c) Irregular hypertrophy of the soft tissues of the nose with enlargement of sebaceous glands, increased vascularity and associated acne.

57 (a) Chronic ectropion of the lower eyelid resulting in epiphora.
(b) Laxity of eyelids is an important mechanism in ectropion. Wedge resection of lower eyelid with application of skin graft is the favoured method of treatment.

58 (a) X-ray of the knee showing loss of joint space and subchondral bony sclerosis—osteoarthritis.
(b) In early cases, the patient experiences pain especially on walking and climbing stairs, with stiffness after a period of immobility. Later the joint loses its full range of flexion and extension. The patient complains of knees 'letting him down' and has recurrent falls. Eventually genu varum deformity may occur. The pain becomes severe and the patient is then completely immobile.
(c) Mild non-specific synovitis.

59 (a) Seborrhoeic wart (basal cell papilloma).
(b) Seborrhoeic warts are easy to diagnose but sometimes they can be confused with solar keratosis, malignant melanoma, lentigo maligna, benign melanocytic naevus, basal cell carcinoma and histiocytoma.

60 (a) Complete heart block.
(b) Most cases of chronic complete heart block unrelated to myocardial infarction or caused by drugs should be treated by permanent artificial pacemaker. In frail, confused or asymptomatic elderly patients sustained release isoprenaline (Saventrine) preparation may relieve heart failure and reduce the frequency of Adams-Stokes attacks and blackouts.

61 (a) Thrombocytopenia, scurvy and metabolic disorders such as uraemia.
(b) Purpura, perifollicular haemorrhages, hyperkeratotic papules, anaemia, bleeding from the gastrointestinal tract, nasal haemorrhage and gum lesions (only in teeth-bearing jaws).

62 (a) Arcus senilis (Gerontoxon).
(b) By lipids being deposited at the periphery of the cornea. There is high incidence in cases of familial hypercholesterolaemias.

63 (a) Right-sided pleural effusion.
(b) Cardiac failure, pneumonia, malignancy, TB, pulmonary infarction and hepatic failure.

64 (a) This is an ophthalmoscopic picture of a small embolus seen as a refractile body filling the lumen of a branch of the retinal artery.
(b) Amaurosis fugax—transient monocular blindness.
(c) Patients may have other features of transient ischaemic attacks in the territory of carotid artery, eg hemiparesis, monoparesis, episodic confusion, unilateral sensory disturbances, dysphasia and hemianopia.

65 (a) Basal cell carcinoma—rodent ulcer.
(b) Rodent ulcers are common in the elderly and there is high incidence with solar irradiation. They can also arise in areas treated by X-rays and from pre-existing naevus sebaceous. Sometimes they are inherited as the basal cell naevus syndrome.

66 (a) Sinus bradycardia, depression of ST segment and flattening of the T waves.
(b) Hypothyroidism.
(c) Cardiomyopathy, cardiac failure and pericardial effusion.

67 (a) Ichthyosis.
(b) Autosomal dominant ichthyosis, sex-linked ichthyosis, ichthyosiform erythroderma and lamellar ichthyosis.
(c) Acquired forms of ichthyosis occur in association with lymphoma, essential fatty acid malabsorption, lipid lowering drugs and leprosy.

68 (a) Hypochromic RBCs, microcytosis and pencil cells.
(b) Iron deficiency anaemia is usually symptomless in early stages. Later the patient experiences lethargy, weakness, tiredness and dizziness. In severe cases cardiac failure may develop and sometimes confusion. There may be associated angular stomatitis or koilonychia. Dysphagia is present in cases of Plummer-Vinson syndrome and recurrent falls are a common presenting feature. Symptoms and signs of underlying pathology usually co-exist.

69 (a) A ring pessary, which has been *in situ* for a long time and probably forgotten. This is a common problem in elderly female patients who may present with urinary incontinence, discomfort or pelvic infection.
(b) The ring pessary should be removed followed by a thorough pelvic examination preferably by a gynaecologist. A vaginal prolapse may need surgery. Co-existing urinary tract infection and vaginitis should be treated by appropriate drugs.

70 (a) Paget's disease of the bone.
(b) The combination of excessive bone breakdown and rapid bone replacement resulting in deformity and increased fragility is characteristic.
(c) Bone aches and pains, mainly in the pelvis and legs. Bone deformities, especially bowing of the tibia and enlargement of the skull, high output cardiac failure, deafness, visual impairment and rarely development of osteogenic sarcoma in the affected bone.

71 (a) Parkinsonism.
(b) Dopamine deficiency in the pigmented nuclei of the brain stem.
(c) Idiopathic Parkinsonism in the elderly is a chronic disease which is progressive. About 60% of the patients die within 10 years of first diagnosis. The causes of death

are bronchopneumonia, pressure sores, urinary tract infections, falls leading to fracture of the femur and other complications of postural instability and wasting.

72 (a) Degenerative changes throughout the cervical spine with loss of normal curvature—cervical spondylosis.
(b) In many elderly people, cervical spine arthritis is without symptoms. However, there is an association with postural imbalance caused by disturbance of cervical articular mechanoreceptor function. Cervical spondylosis frequently co-exists with vertebrobasilar insufficiency. *Other clinical features include:* brachial radiculitis—pain and paraesthesiae; headaches, giddiness and falls; drop attacks; diplopia; facial sensory disturbances; dysarthria; weakness of legs and unsteadiness; paraplegia or quadriplegia in severe cases.

73 (a) Paget's disease (osteitis deformans).
(b) If simple analgesics fail then calcitonin is used for severe bone pain. Salmon calcitonin is given in doses of 100 MRC units three times weekly by subcutaneous injection for up to six months. Diphosphonates and Mithranycin can also be used but are less effective. Pain due to associated osteoarthrosis is treated with physiotherapy, heat treatment and NSAIDs.

74 (a) Acromegaly is due to hypersecretion of growth hormone by acidophil cells after the epiphyses have united. Excess growth hormone production is usually due to an acidophil macroadenoma of the pituitary.
(b) The skin becomes thick and coarse and there is increase in the size of subcutaneous tissues. Enlargement of the tongue, lips, nose and ears is obvious. There is also enlargement of supraorbital ridges, sinuses and lower jaw.

75 (a) Glossitis.
(b) Loss of teeth, ill-fitting dentures, denture hyperplasia and denture stomatitis, atrophic glossitis, reduced mucus secretion, varicosity of the mucosal vessels on the underside of the tongue, hyperkeratotic lesions of the oral mucosa, xerostomia and reduced taste sensation.

76 (a) Subluxation of the left shoulder joint.
(b) Left hemiplegia.
(c) Painful frozen shoulder.

77 (a) Steroid purpura.
(b) Thinning, striae, easy bruising, poor wound healing, acne and hypertrichosis.
(c) Euphoria, psychosis, increased intracranial pressure and myopathy.

78 (a) Typical linear deposits of calcium pyrophosphate in the menisci and articular cartilage with some degenerative changes similar to osteoarthritis.
(b) Examination of the joint aspirate by polarizing microscopy will reveal the typical intraleucocytic positively birefringent crystals of calcium pyrophosphate dihydrate.

79 (a) Pressure sores are common in elderly patients who are paralysed, immobile or unconscious. Compression and shearing forces act in cases where there is poor tissue perfusion, immobility, paresis, malnutrition, anaemias, carcinomas, hypoxaemia and urinary incontinence.
(b) Treating the underlying condition and avoiding immobility or pressure over the bony prominences. Regular turning and meticulous nursing care of the pressure points on the body are required. A variety of beds and bedding are available, eg sheepskin underblankets, ripple beds, air beds. Desloughing agents are used to clean sores and various types of dressings are available which promote moist tissue healing.

80 (a) Constipation leading to faecal impaction. The patient had been trying to clear his rectum with his hands.
(b) Severe faecal impaction may require manual clearance. In other cases a series of enemas may suffice. Plain X-ray of the abdomen will show constipated faeces higher up in the colon and for this the patient will need laxatives and a high-fibre diet. Faecal impaction is a frequent cause of acute toxic confusion in the elderly.

81 (a) Anterior myocardial infarction.
(b) Rapidly increasing dyspnoea in 20%, chest pain in 20%, acute confusional states, syncope, hemiplegia due to embolic cerebral infarction, embolic occlusion of non-cerebral arteries, renal failure, vomiting and intense weakness.

82 (a) Goitre.
(b) Simple goitre, Hashimoto's thyroiditis, subacute (de Quervain's) thyroiditis, drug-induced goitre, and malignant and benign tumours of thyroid.

83 (a) Miliary tuberculosis.
(b) Lassitude and exhaustion, loss of weight and anaemia are common initial symptoms. Respiratory symptoms are less frequent and the characteristic miliary shadows on chest X-rays may be absent. In a minority of patients there is pyrexia, attacks of sweating, tachycardia, anaemia, rapid weight loss, cough and dyspnoea.

84 (a) Osteoarthritis of the shoulder.
(b) Pain and stiffness of the shoulder with associated weakness of the arm.
(c) Supraspinatus tendinitis, subacromial bursitis, traumatic lesions of the rotator cuff, capsulitis, subluxation, fractures and shoulder-hand syndrome.

85 (a) The outstanding feature is the marked proliferation of abnormal melanocytic cells in the junctional zone. The abnormal cells extend upwards, laterally and downwards. A tumour depth of 2.5 mm or more indicates a poor prognosis.
(b) Itching, inflammation, increase in size and change of shape, variation in colour, surface breakdown and bleeding.

86 (a) Multiple fluid levels in a case of intestinal obstruction.
(b) Severe constipation, adhesions from old operations, carcinoma colon, ischaemic colitis, hypokalaemia and hypercalcaemia.

87 (a) There is loss of articular cartilage and small cystic areas in the head and neck of the femur. Subchondral bone has areas of sclerosis and protrusio acetabuli is in development—a case of advanced osteoarthritis.
(b) Simple analgesics and then NSAIDs to relieve pain; surgery in severe cases (total hip replacement); and general measures—weight reduction, walking stick or walking frame, physiotherapy to maintain muscle power and range of movement and hydrotherapy for painful and stiff hips.

88 (a) By checking liver function tests, plain X-ray of the abdomen, isotope scan of the liver, abdominal ultrasound, endoscopy and, if necessary, CT scanning.
(b) Congestive cardiac failure, hepatic metastases, myeloproliferative disorders, biliary obstruction and cirrhosis of the liver.

89 (a) Spinal kyphosis, most probably due to osteoporosis.
(b) Chronic back pain, reduced mobility, inability to recline comfortably in the bed, interference with pulmonary function, abdominal discomfort and risk of pressure sores developing over bony prominences of the spine.

90 (a) Acrosclerosis in systemic sclerosis; fingers shiny and tapered.
(b) Raynaud's phenomenon is present in 80-90% of the patients.
(c) The basic pathological abnormality of this multisystem inflammatory disorder is deposition of new collagen and/or an obliterative vasculitis in affected areas.

91 (a) Motor neurone disease.
(b) Amyotrophic lateral sclerosis, progressive bulbar palsy, and progressive muscular atrophy.
(c) Conditions that mimic motor neurone disease are systematized motor neurone lesions of carcinoma bronchus, diabetic amyotrophy, meningovascular syphilis and cervical spondylosis.

92 (a) Diabetes, myxoedema, hepatic failure, chronic renal failure, lymphoma, reticulosis, carcinomatosis, psychological, carcinoma lung and drugs eg alkaloids.
(b) Scabies, pediculosis, eczema, urticaria, lichen planus, dermatitis herpetiformis, lichen simplex chronicus and ichthyosis.

93 (a) Diverticular disease of the colon.
(b) Usually asymptomatic. Pain in the left iliac fossa in 78%, constipation in 35%, diarrhoea in 19%, flatulence in 13%, rectal bleeding in 30%, nausea and loss of appetite.
(c) Diverticulosis, haemorrhage, anaemia, abscess formation and perforation leading to peritonitis, pericolic abscess and fistula formation into other viscera.

94 (a) Herpes simplex (herpes febrilis).
(b) Keep the affected area clean and dry and treat the underlying condition eg chest infection. If the attack of herpes is severe and painful, then topical acyclovir may be helpful in reducing the symptoms.

95 (a) Subcapital fracture of the neck of the femur.
(b) Fall or sudden mechanical stress in a patient who has osteoporosis, osteomalacia, Paget's disease or bony metastases.
(c) Subcapital, transcervical, intertrochanteric and subtrochanteric.

96 (a) Calcification, most probably in the thyroid.
(b) X-ray of the neck and thoracic inlet will show any significant goitre, whether it is compressing the trachea or if there is any retrosternal extension. Ultrasonography will differentiate between purely cystic (benign) and partially cystic (malignant?) adenomas. Examination of the vocal cords will show if there is damage to recurrent laryngeal nerve. High serum autoantibodies to the thyroid are indicative of Hashimoto's thyroiditis. If the nature of goitre is still in doubt then needle biopsy of the thyroid is indicated.

97 (a) Gaseous distension of the stomach.
(b) Abdominal discomfort or pain, anorexia, hiccoughs, nausea, vomiting and features of dehydration and metabolic upset.
(c) Fibre optic gastroscopy.

98 (a) Eczema craquelé (xerosis).
(b) Low relative humidity tends to dry out the horny layer of the skin causing chaffing, xerosis and itchiness. When the cold conditions are compounded by repeated washing, a form of eczema appears which is prominent on the legs. Its typical pattern is like crazy paving.

99 (a) Sebaceous gland hyperplasia.
(b) Nodular basal cell carcinoma.

100 (a) Shadow containing an air bubble behind the cardiac silhouette—hiatus hernia.
(b) Usually it produces no symptoms and is an accidental finding on an X-ray done for some other reason. However, clinical features can be divided into three groups: *symptoms caused by oesophagitis*—dysphagia, discomfort in chest with bending, stooping or lying down, and angina-like chest pains; *symptoms caused by hernia*—retrosternal discomfort and irritation of diaphragm causing cough and hiccoughs; *symptoms caused by haemorrhage*—chronic blood loss leading to

anaemia, rapid blood loss may result in shock. Associated oesophagitis may eventually result in development of a stricture which will cause dysphagia.

101 (a) Bell-shaped thorax in a case of osteomalacia and/or osteoporosis.
(b) Serum calcium, inorganic phosphate and alkaline phosphatase estimations. Further X-rays to check for pseudofractures and compression fractures of the vertebrae. Isotope bone scan will show focal hot areas of increased uptake in cases of osteomalacia. Bone biopsy will distinguish between osteomalacia and osteoporosis. Patients with osteomalacia will respond dramatically to a therapeutic trial of vitamin D.

102 (a) Calcification of aortic knuckle. This is a benign condition associated with advancing age, atheroma and aortic sclerosis.
(b) Calcified syphilitic aortitis and calcified aortic aneurysms.

103 (a) In the right third cranial nerve.
(b) Third cranial nerve may be involved in multiple sclerosis, meningovascular syphilis, diabetes mellitus, cerebral aneurysms and other intracerebral space occupying lesions.

104 (a) Squamous cell carcinoma.
(b) This is a common skin neoplasm in the elderly occurring on sun damaged skin. Heat injury can also provoke its development. It can also arise from areas treated by X-rays and from pre-existing skin lesions including chronic discoid lupus erythematosus, lupus vulgaris, chronic varicose ulcers, warty naevi and genital warts.
(c) Small lesions should be excised completely with a 3-5 mm margin. Radiotherapy is effective but may leave fragile scars. Cryotherapy or topical Fluorouracil can also be used with success.

105 (a) Facial cyanosis.
(b) FEV1 will be reduced and the ratio of FEV1 to vital capacity is also low. The residual volume will be increased at the expense of vital capacity. The PaO_2 falls will be normal and there may be sustained rise in $PaCO_2$. In some patients there may be impairment of gas transfer also.

106 (a) Reflux oesophagitis.
(b) The patient should be advised to adopt measures to reduce reflux. Meals should be small and fatty food should be avoided. Weight reduction is essential. Do not stoop or bend. At night the patient should sleep with the head end of the bed elevated. Smoking should be stopped or reduced. Non steroidal anti-inflammatory drugs should be stopped or reduced. Heartburn can be relieved by antacids taken frequently through the day. Cimetidine or Ranitidine given over a period of time may result in healing of oesophagitis. Patients with strictures will require liquid or semi-liquid diet and if necessary endoscopic dilatation. If severe symptoms persist, despite adequate medical therapy, then surgical resection of the stricture is indicated in selected patients.

107 (a) Dental caries and periodontal (gum) disease.
(b) Inability to chew food properly, malnourishment and anaemia, stomatitis and mouth ulcers, candidosis and, in susceptible patients, septicaemia and bacterial endocarditis.

108 (a) Thickening and hypertrophy of the nail plate.
(b) Psoriasis and onychomycosis.

109 (a) Intertriginous dermatitis.
(b) This is common in obese patients with poor personal hygiene. Sweating encourages microbial growth on the skin surfaces and large pendulous folds of skin exaggerate these effects. *Candida albicans* is often found in such lesions and some

patients may also complain of urinary incontinence.

110 (a) Pulmonary metastases.
(b) Renal carcinoma (hypernephroma).
(c) Renal colic due to haematuria and blood clots, PUO, metastases in liver and lung, polycythaemia. The tumour may be palpable.

111 (a) The incidence of falls increases linearly with age and they are more common in women. They tend to occur indoors and often happen when the patient is moving from bed, wheelchair or the toilet. There is also increased incidence in people who are socially isolated, depressed or demented.
(b) Common complications are: fractures, especially neck of femur and wrist; head injury and sometimes subdural haematoma; hypothermia; burns; dehydration; bronchopneumonia; depression; loss of confidence; immobility.

112 (a) Rectal examination.
(b) Faecal lumps in the rectum and colon—constipation.
(c) Reduced dietary intake of fibre and roughage; lack of exercise and immobility; poor bowel habits; lack of privacy, eg in hospitals, and difficulty in adapting to new environment; drugs—codeine, antidepressants, iron salts, anticholinergics; colonic lesions—diverticular disease of the colon, CA colon, idiopathic megacolon, spastic colon, obstruction; anal lesions—fissures, abscess, piles.

113 (a) Convexed meningioma.
(b) Vague psychiatric disorders—apathy, reduced social awareness, deterioration of memory, dementia and incontinence; also fist and grasp reflex in the contralateral hand; olfactory nerve involvement leading to unilateral loss of sense of smell; general features due to increased intracranial pressure—headaches drowsiness, fits, dizziness, papilloedema, vomiting, bradycardia, hypertension and false localizing signs.

114 (a) Contracture—caused by spasticity resulting from old hemiplegia, ulnar nerve palsy or Dupuytren's contracture.
(b) Early physiotherapy and gradually increasing doses of anti-spasticity drugs such as Dantrolene and Baclofen.

115 (a) Calcification in the wall of ascending aorta—due to syphilitic aortitis.
(b) Congenital bicuspid valves, rheumatic heart disease, infected endocarditis, cystic medial necrosis, Marfan's syndrome, ankylosing spondylitis, atheroma and late syphilis.

116 (a) Areas of pulmonary fibrosis—'shaggy' appearance of the left heart border.
(b) (1) fibrosing alveolitis; (2) pleural effusions and pleuritis; (3) nodules in lungs or pleura; (4) Caplan's syndrome with pneumoconiosis; (5) increased incidence of small airways obstruction in smokers; (6) acute pneumonitis (rare).

117 (a) Hemiplegic oedema of the right hand. This is non-pitting oedema and is due to a combination of muscle paralysis, disuse and autonomic changes.
(b) Physiotherapy and exercises. Arm elevation, gentle compression by inflatable splint. Diuretics are of very little benefit.

118 (a) Infiltration with atypical plasma cells—a case of multiple myeloma.
(b) There is excessive production of paraprotein which is lost in the urine as Bence-Jones protein. This blocks the renal tubules resulting in renal damage. Renal failure may also be due to amyloidosis and hypercalcaemia causing nephrocalcinosis.

119 (a) Aneurysm involving the descending aorta.
(b) Aneurysms of aorta are usually due to atherosclerosis and hypertension, but some cases are due to cystic medial necrosis, syphilis and non-penetrating chest trauma.

120 (a) Wasting of the small muscles of the hand.
(b) The likely causes are: (1) cord lesions—tumours, eg meningioma, motor neurone disease, cord compression, trauma, vascular lesions; (2) root lesions, eg cervical spondylosis; (3) brachial plexus lesions—cervical rib, Pancoast's tumour; (4) nerve lesions—carpal tunnel syndrome, ulnar nerve lesion, polyneuropathy; (5) miscellaneous—shoulder-hand syndrome, rheumatoid arthritis, disuse atrophy.

121 (a) Glabellar tap—blinking provoked by tapping the glabella repeatedly does not show the normal habituation.
(b) Parkinsonism, cerebral atrophy, Alzheimer's dementia, arteriosclerotic dementia and progressive supranuclear palsy.

122 (a) Sclerosis of the vertebral body.
(b) The sclerotic appearance of the vertebra is usually due to metastases and this is commonly from CA prostate, breast or lung. This patient will need rectal and breast examination, estimation of acid phosphatase, chest X-ray and radiological survey of the skeleton.

123 (a) Heberden's nodes—bony swellings in the distal interphalangeal joints.
(b) Osteoarthritis.
(c) Pain in one or more joints, worst towards the evening, and increased by particular activity. 80% of patients have morning stiffness. Other symptoms are reduced mobility, associated obesity, depression, falls and insomnia.

124 (a) Bronchopneumonia.
(b) In some cases the symptoms and signs may not be immediately referrable to the chest. Patients present with general deterioration, falls, confusion, cough, dyspnoea, chest pains, tachycardia and tachypnoea. On auscultation the air entry is poor and coarse crackles are heard over both lung fields. Pyrexia and leucocytosis are unusual.

125 (a) Hyperostosis frontalis interna.
(b) None—this is a benign radiological condition discovered accidentally in the elderly.
(c) It may be confused with Paget's disease, multiple myeloma, osteoporosis circumscripta, fractures of the skull and meningioma.

126 (a) Side view of a fixed brain showing shrunken gyri and gaping sulci. There is extreme shrinkage of the temporal lobe as well as generalized cerebral atrophy, more marked anteriorly.
(b) The clinical features will be those of senile dementia, very slow in progression and deterioration: forgetfulness, nocturnal agitation, deteriorating habits, difficulty with activities of daily living, especially handling money; patient is faulted on current events and time; then confusional episodes and disorientation leading to deterioration of personal care and hygiene; incorrect responses; antisocial behaviour; eventually complete incapacity to look after self.

127 (a) Contralateral hemiplegia, sensory loss, motor aphasia and hemianopia.
(b) Unconsciousness, old age, hypertension, confusion or dementia, unequal pupils, Cheyne-Stokes breathing, bilateral CNS signs, 2nd or 3rd stroke and chest infection.

128 (a) Figurate or annular erythema.
(b) Persistent or recurrent skin eruption of this kind indicates internal malignancy, especially carcinoma bronchus.
(c) Hyperpigmentation, pallor, pruritus, acanthosis nigricans, dermatomyositis, herpes zoster, acquired ichthyosis, figurate erythema, superficial migratory thrombophlebitis, pemphigoid, generalized hyperhidrosis. The skin may also be directly involved by internal malignant disease.

129 (a) Plaques of psoriasis.

(b) Family history, onset following an episode of stress, lesions appearing at sites of minor trauma (Kobner phenomenon), lesions improving after exposure to sunlight, lack of itching, and presence of associated arthritis.

(b) Guttate psoriasis, pustular lesions, flexural psoriasis, napkin psoriasis in children, generalized pustular psoriasis and erythrodermic psoriasis.

130 (a) Bouchard's nodes—a feature of osteoarthritis similar to Heberden's nodes but occurring in the proximal interphalangeal joints.

(b) (1) Congenital structural abnormalities, eg hypermobility; (2) structural childhood disorders, eg Perthes' disease, slipped femoral epiphysis; (3) trauma and mechanical problems, eg meniscectomy and recurrent dislocation; (4) crystal deposition disease, eg pyrophosphate arthropathy and gout; (5) metabolic abnormalities, eg ochronosis; (6) avascular necrosis; (7) septic arthritis and recurrent haemarthrosis in haemophilia.

131 (a) Caput medusae.

(b) Formation of portal-systemic collateral circulation due to portal hypertension.

(c) Sites of collateral circulation: in the distal oesophagus and proximal stomach; in the anus and distal rectum; in the falciform ligament and between the colonic omental splenic and retroperitoneal veins. Collateral vessels appearing on the anterior abdominal wall and radiating from the umbilicus are called Caput medusae.

132 (a) The approximate incidence is 190 per 100,000 per year in females.

(b) Radiological examination of the chest and skeleton. Radioisotope scanning of the liver and spine is a good method of detecting small metastases. Confirmation of the diagnosis by histological examination of biopsy material should always be obtained.

133 (a) The X-ray shows osteoporotic spine with increased translucency of the vertebral bodies and wedging and impaction fractures of the brittle mid thoracic vertebrae.

(b) The aetiology of osteoporosis in the elderly is complex. The main factors are: (1) post-menopausal bone loss in females; (2) poor skeletal development of females; (3) prolonged negative calcium balance in some individuals; (4) nutritional factors—deficiencies of calcium, vitamin D, vitamin C, protein and fluoride—also post-gastrectomy and malabsorption; (5) prolonged immobilization; (6) hyperadrenocorticism; (7) hyperthyroidism; (8) acromegaly; (9) rheumatoid arthritis.

134 (a) Neurofibrillary tangle is composed of thick strands of argentophilic material filling the neuronal cytoplasm and extending into apical dendrite.

(b) Senile dementia (Alzheimer's disease) and multi-infarct dementia are the two most common types. Chronic dementia also occurs in Huntington's chorea, advanced Parkinsonism, Jakob-Creutzfeldt disease, Pick's disease and multiple sclerosis.

135 (a) Scald, carpet burn, pressure sore.

(b) Silent myocardial infarction, arrhythmias, heart block, postural hypotension, subclavian steal syndrome, anaemia, carotid sinus hypersensitivity and vertebrobasilar insufficiency.

136 (a) Osteoporosis—reduction of both protein matrix and mineralization.

(b) Osteoporosis is usually asymptomatic. A common symptom is backache caused by vertebral collapse. Fracture of the neck of the femur and Colles' fracture are frequent presenting signs. Some patients experience symptoms of nerve root compression and increasing kyphoscoliosis with loss of height and deteriorating mobility.

137 (a) Post-herpetic neuralgia and depression, secondary bacterial infection, ophthalmic herpes zoster, Ramsay-Hunt syndrome (herpes of geniculate ganglion resulting in severe facial palsy and vesicular eruption in external auditory canal), encephalitis and generalized herpes zoster.
(b) The affected area needs frequent cleaning with saline or a weak antiseptic solution. Analgesics are required to relieve pain. Prednisolone given early reduces the risk of post-herpetic neuralgia. Prednisolone 60 mg daily is given for 2-4 weeks and then gradually reduced. Acyclovir given IV or by mouth in early stages of disease reduces the severity and duration and should be used in frail elderly patients.

138 (a) Ruptured abdominal aortic aneurysm with features of advanced atheroma.
(b) With abdominal pain and features of acute abdomen and shock.

139 (a) Hypersegmented neutrophils and oval macrocytes.
(b) Vitamin B12 and/or folate deficiency. *The causes of vitamin B12 deficiency* are poor diet, pernicious anaemia, atrophic gastritis, gastrectomy, carcinoma stomach, malabsorption, ileal resection. *The causes of folic deficiency* are poor diet and malabsorption, chronic diseases, neoplasm, liver disease, drugs, eg Phenytoin.
(c) Non-specific signs of anaemia, yellow tinge to the skin in pernicious anaemia, anorexia, glossitis, peripheral neuropathy, sub-acute combined degeneration, mild confusion, depression and dementia.

140 (a) Central retinal artery thrombosis.
(b) Acute glaucoma, retinal detachment, vitreous haemorrhage, thrombosis or embolism of retinal artery, thrombosis of retinal vein, cranial arteritis and cerebral infarct or haemorrhage.

141 (a) Carcinoma lung.
(b) Inappropriate ADH production—hyponatraemia; parathormone production—hypercalcaemia; ectopic ACTH production—hypokalaemic alkalosis, weakness, oedema, diabetes and hyperpigmentation; carcinoid syndrome; thyrotoxicosis; hypoglycaemic episodes; gynaecomastia; red cell aplasia.

142 (a) Right-sided ptosis.
(b) Congenital, oculomotor nerve lesions, cervical sympathetic lesion (Horner's), myasthenia gravis, myopathy, tabes dorsalis, multiple sclerosis, senile ptosis, corticosteroid-induced ptosis.
(c) Pupillary constriction, enophthalmos, ptosis and impaired sweating on that side of the face.

143 (a) Vaginal prolapse.
(b) Trabeculation and formation of cellules or pseudodiverticula and diverticula.
(c) Uninhibited neurogenic bladder, eg dementias, strokes, parietal and frontal lobe lesions; Reflex neurogenic bladder—paraplegia; retention with overflow—tabes, diabetes and prostatism; Autonomous bladder—cauda equina lesions.

144 (a) Four reasons: (1) they often live in cold houses; (2) reduced sensitivity to cold; (3) impairment of thermoregulatory mechanism. They respond poorly to cold temperature, ie by putting on extra clothes, lighting the fire, etc; (4) inability to increase heat production by shivering and to conserve heat by cutaneous vasoconstriction.
(b) Bronchopneumonia, intravascular thrombosis causing stroke, myocardial infarction, mesenteric occlusion and peripheral gangrene, pancreatitis, pressure sores, hypoglycaemia.

145 (a) Nikolsky sign—rubbing apparently normal skin causes the superficial epidermis to slough off.

(b) There is characteristic cell splitting within the epidermal layer called acantholysis. There is also deposition of immunoglobulin in the epidermal intercellular spaces.

(c) Pemphigus vulgaris; pemphigoid; Stevens-Johnson syndrome; drug reactions.

146 (a) Atrial fibrillation.

(b) Ischaemic heart disease, hypertension, mitral valvular disease, myocardial infarction, pericarditis, aortic valvular disease, thyrotoxicosis, lone atrial fibrillation, sick sinus syndrome and infections, eg bronchopneumonia.

147 (a) Pitting and ridging of the nails—psoriasis.

(b) Psoriatic arthropathy commonly affects the distal interphalangeal joints and is usually asymmetrical. It is seronegative and rheumatoid nodules are absent. 10% develop arthropathy, 30% give history of psoriasis. There are four main patterns: distal type 55%; seronegative type but indistinguishable from rheumatoid arthritis; deforming type; and spondylitis.

148 (a) Median nerve (carpal tunnel syndrome).

(b) Pronators of the forearm, long finger flexors and abductors and opponens muscles of the thumb.

(c) By nerve conduction studies, which show motor and sensory impairment across the carpal tunnel.

149 (a) Lupus erythematosus.

(b) 'Butterfly' eruption over the face, photosensitivity, discoid lesions, alopecia, vasculitis.

(c) Patients in the 6th decade account for about 12% of those with systemic lupus erythematosus. In the elderly there is higher frequency of pericarditis, pulmonary abnormalities, arthritis and skin lesions. Renal disease, Raynaud's phenomenon and neuropsychiatric disorders are less frequent.

150 (a) Several areas of cerebral infarction.

(b) Multiple infarct dementia.

(c) The patient, usually an elderly man, suffers step-wise deterioration of both physical and mental health. Clinical features include weakness, slowness, depression, dysarthria, dysphagia, small-stepped gait, brisk tendon jerks and rigid limbs. Pseudobulbar palsy may develop. Memory fails and there is pathological laughing and crying. Self-neglect, perseveration, incontinence, paranoid symptoms and immobility appear over a period of time.

151 (a) Cellulitis.

(b) Deep vein thrombosis and superficial thrombophlebitis.

(c) Analgesics, rest, leg elevation and broad spectrum antibiotics.

152 (a) Intracerebral haemorrhage.

(b) This occurs with sudden onset of severe headache, vomiting and unconsciousness. There may be signs of meningism and periodic breathing. Frequently there is involvement of internal capsule giving rise to a dense hemiplegia and hemianaesthesia.

153 (a) Bacterial endocarditis.

(b) *Streptococcus viridans* is still the commonest but relatively less than before—still over 50%.

(c) In 1945, 18% of the patients over 60 years, now 25% over 60 years. Prognosis is usually poor with mortality of about 70% and this condition often occurs as a terminal illness. The underlying heart disease is less often rheumatic mitral disease and more frequently aortic valve disease of uncertain origin.

154 (a) Tophaceous gout.
(b) Myeloproliferative disorders, eg polycythaemia rubra vera during treatment of malignant disease; renal failure, eg due to lead poisoning; hypothyroidism; Lesch-Nyhan syndrome; glycogen storage disease; drugs, eg diuretics.

155 (a) Xanthelasmas.
(b) Hyperlipidaemia (hypercholesterolaemia).
(c) Ischaemic heart disease.

156 (a) A space occupying lesion involving most of the right parietal lobe, probably glioma.
(b) Jacksonian epilepsy of sensory type, difficulty in localizing sensations on the opposite side of body, spatial disorientation, aproxia, agnosia, perceptual rivalry, receptive dysphasia (lesions on the dominant side), homonymous hemianopia.

157 (a) Keratoconjunctivitis.
(b) Adenovirus.

158 (a) *Streptococcus pneumoniae, Staphylococcus aureus, Streptococcus pyogenes, Klebsiella pneumoniae, H. influenzae, Legionella pneumophila, Mycoplasma, Coxiella burnetii,* psittacosis and ornithosis, influenza virus.
(b) Fever and toxaemia appear early. Severe headache, weakness and anorexia. Physical signs in the chest appear late and are mild. Occasionally there is splenomegaly and the white cell count is normal.

159 (a) Bone metastases.
(b) Adequate 24-hour pain control, attention to nutrition, bowels and bladder, counselling by a specialist nurse or doctor, radiotherapy in selected cases, treatment of hypercalcaemia, sympathetic nursing and, if possible, treatment of the underlying disorder.

160 (a) Lipodermatosclerosis—varicose eczema associated with chronic venous insufficiency.
(b) Lack of venous drainage in the leg due to incompetent venous valves between the superficial veins and the larger deep veins with reversal of blood flow—from deep to superficial veins—causing rise of pressure in the superficial veins which results in stasis, oedema, ulcers and eczema. Incompetent valves occur due to deep vein thrombosis, primary long saphenous vein insufficiency, familial venous valve incompetence and deep venous obstruction. Ulcers occur because of oedema in the subcutaneous tissues with poor lymphatic and capillary drainage and extra vascular accumulation of fibrinous material that has leaked from the blood vessels causing rigid cuffs around the capillaries preventing diffusion through the wall and fibrosis of the surrounding tissue.

161 (a) Chronic venous insufficiency, deep vein thrombosis, deep venous obstruction, obesity, peripheral arterial atheroma, vasculitis, arterial obstruction, eg rheumatoid arthritis and collagen diseases, hypertension, diabetes, ulcerative colitis, malignant disease, eg squamous cell carcinoma, basal cell carcinoma, melanoma, Kaposi's sarcoma, trauma and infections.
(b) Arterial ulcers have clear cut edges and are accompanied by pain which is usually worse at night. The pretibial area is affected rather than the ankle. Phlebography and Doppler ultrasound may help in distinguishing between arterial and venous ulcers.

162 (a) Cataract.
(b) Glaucoma, ophthalmitis, degenerative myopia, retinal detachment, trauma and irradiation.

163 (a) Unequal pupils.

(b) Lesions of the third cranial nerve and cervical sympathetic chain.

164 (a) Incisional hernia.
(b) Abdominal pain and discomfort, loss of confidence, constipation and intestinal obstruction.

165 (a) Ectopic ACTH syndrome, hypoadrenalism, acromegaly, hyperthyroidism, pheochromocytoma.
(b) Jaundice; carotenaemia; haemosiderosis.

166 (a) Scabies.
(b) The characteristic distribution involves the fingers, wrists, nipples, abdomen, genitalia, buttocks and ankles. It does not occur above the neck.
(c) Gamma benzene hexachloride and 25% benzyl benzoate emulsion.

167 (a) Raynaud's phenomenon.
(b) Paroxysmal digital ischaemia, with pallor and cyanosis followed by erythema.
(c) (1) Raynaud's disease; (2) cervical spondylosis; (3) use of vibrating machinery; (4) arteriosclerosis; (5) Buerger's disease; (6) systemic sclerosis; (7) dysproteinaemias; (8) cold agglutinins; (9) polycythaemia; (10) cold injury.

168 (a) Oculogyric crisis—sustained involuntary and conjugate deviation of the eyes upward.
(b) Post-encephalitic and drug-induced Parkinsonism.

169 (a) Hypokalaemia—note the U waves.
(b) (1) Weakness of skeletal muscles; (2) constipation and ileus; (3) cardiac arrhythmias; (4) paraesthesiae; (5) apathy and confusion.

170 (a) Atypical lymphocytes showing chronic lymphatic leukaemia.
(b) It becomes increasing infiltrated with lymphocytes whose antibody formation function is abnormal.

171 (a) Intense erythema and telangiectasia.
(b) Chronic exposure of the skin to ultraviolet radiation from the sun.

172 (a) Lentigo.
(b) Chronic solar exposure.
(c) Lentigo maligna and malignant melanoma.

173 (a) Interstitial pulmonary fibrosis.
(b) Gas transfer defect with maldistribution of pulmonary ventilation and perfusion leading to hypoxaemia, hyperventilation and hypocapnia.
(c) Coal dust, silica, asbestos, talc, iron oxide, aluminium, china clay, tin dioxide and beryllium.

174 (a) Filling defect in the bladder and hydronephrosis.
(b) (1) Haematuria; (2) bile; (3) increased concentration; (4) porphyria; (5) myoglobinuria.

175 (a) Calcified costochondral cartilages.
(b) None.

176 (a) Multiple pulmonary emboli.
(b) Dyspnoea, pleural pain, tachycardia, haemoptysis, syncope, central cyanosis and pyrexia. Sometimes pulmonary infarction is symptomless.

177 (a) Puffiness below the eyes.
(b) Nephrotic syndrome.
(c) Angio-oedema, myxoedema and corticosteroid therapy.

178 (a) (1) Ovarian neoplasm; (2) obesity; (3) ascites; (4) mesenteric cyst; (5) retroperitoneal tumours.
(b) Epithelial tumours 70-80%; stromal origin tumours 10%; germ cell tumours 5%; other groups.
(c) Torsion of the pedicle, haemorrhage, rupture, degeneration, infection, malignant change and intestinal obstruction.

179 (a) Lymphoedema.
(b) Carcinoma breast.
(c) Mammography, xerography and thermography.

180 (a) Solar keratosis.
(b) Chronic damage from solar ultraviolet radiation and, rarely, erythema ab igne and chronic arsenic poisoning.

181 (a) Tobacco staining, food and chromogenic organisms.
(b) Due to elongation of filiform papillae of the medial dorsal surface area caused by failure of keratin layer of the papillae to desquamate normally, plus growth of chromogenic organisms.

182 (a) Sick sinus syndrome is a condition in which abnormal node function may be associated with other abnormalities in the conducting system. The most common arrhythmia is the bradycardia-tachycardia syndrome which is characterized by recurrent supraventricular tachycardia in patients who have sinus bradycardia.
(b) Patient may be asymptomatic but in the elderly it may present with palpitations, dizziness, falls and blackouts.

183 (a) Polymyalgia rheumatica.
(b) High ESR, normochromic, normocytic anaemia. Temporal artery biopsy shows giant cell arteritis in 40% of the patients.
(c) The natural history is for remission to occur in six months to 2 years although relapses are not uncommon.

184 (a) Advanced changes with papilloedema, haemorrhages and exudates.
(b) Hypertensives develop 4-7 times as many strokes as normotensives.
(c) The treatment of hypertension in the elderly remains controversial but some general guidelines are as follows: (1) take several readings before diagnosing hypertension; (2) treat systolic BP over 180 mm/Hg and diastolic BP over 110 mm/Hg; (3) consider treatment in the light of known risk factors; (4) reduce BP gradually; (5) check BP lying and standing to detect postural hypotension; (6) treat over 80 year old patients only if there are complications such as left ventricular failure; (7) bear in mind quality of life, mental state, co-existing disabilities and drug compliance.

185 (a) Peroneal nerve.
(b) Peroneal nerve palsy as a result of prolonged pressure over the head of the fibula due to immobility.

186 (a) Alteration of the oral anatomy due to paresis.
(b) Inability to chew food, malnutrition, stomatitis and gum ulcers, drooling of saliva.

187 (a) This is a condition in which there is adhesive capsulitis but little or no synovitis. The pain is often worse at night.
(b) None. The X-ray is usually normal unless there is some other associated disease or disuse osteoporosis.

188 (a) Sensory and social deprivation, withdrawal, depression, slow responses, agitation and being labelled as demented.

(b) Presbycusis, wax in external auditory canal, perforation of tympanic membrane, otosclerosis, Menière's disease, herpes zoster infection, acoustic neuroma, drugs, eg Neomycin, Frusemide.

189 (a) Inflammatory cell infiltration in the arterial wall with multinucleate giant cells—temporal arteritis.
(b) Anorexia, weight loss, headaches, hyperalgesia of scalp, the temporal artery may be thickened, tender and non-pulsating, pain on chewing, neck stiffness, blurred vision leading to loss of vision, co-existing polymyalgia rheumatica, fundi may show ischaemic papillopathy or central retinal artery occlusion.

190 (a) Senile (disciform) macular degeneration.
(b) Coarse dark mottling around the macula.

191 (a) Plaques of pleural calcification on the left side.
(b) Pleural plaques, benign pleural effusion with pain, fever and leucocytosis, pulmonary asbestosis with dyspnoea, mottling and sometimes honeycombing of the lungs and mesothelioma of the pleura.

192 (a) There are four main causes of transient urinary incontinence: (1) infective—urinary tract infection; (2) retention with overflow—faecal impaction, anticholinergic drugs; (3) increased diuresis—diuretics, diabetes mellitus; (4) toxic confusional states, oversedation and psychological.
(b) Mainly infection of the bladder and kidneys. Also septicaemia, loss of confidence, depression and social isolation.

193 (a) Looser's zone (pseudofracture) in the upper tibia.
(b) Osteomalacia.
(c) Vitamin D deficiency.

194 (a) Disseminated intravascular coagulation.
(b) Amniotic fluid embolism, abruptio placentae, eclampsia, dead fetus in utero, malignancies, hepatic disease, severe trauma, anaphylaxis, hypoxia, venoms and sepsis.

195 (a) Congestive cardiac failure.
(b) Obstruction to venous return in the left innominate vein by an elongated and unfolded aorta and superior mediastinal obstruction.

196 (a) Parotid gland.
(b) Mixed parotid tumour; parotitis; sarcoidosis.

197 (a) Localized areas of depigmentation due to vitiligo.
(b) Thyroid disease, pernicious anaemia, hyperparathyroidism, Addison's disease, diabetes mellitus, myasthenia gravis and alopecia areata.

198 (a) Seborrhoeic dermatitis.
(b) (1) Pityriasis capitis; (2) neurodermatitis; (3) pediculosis; (4) lupus erythematosus; (5) contact dermatitis.

199 (a) Osteoarthritis of the knee and calcification of the popliteal artery.
(b) No, apart from the fact that they are both common in the elderly.

200 (a) Spasticity of the hand due to hemiplegia.
(b) There are several different methods of treatment but currently the most popular method is that of Bobath—a form of rehabilitation in which the aim is to change abnormal patterns of posture and movements and reduce spasticity by using key points of control.

INDEX

Numbers refer not to pages but to the number shared by the illustration, question and answer.

Animal studies have demonstrated that felodipine crosses the blood-brain barrier and the placenta.

Cardiovascular Effects

Following administration of PLENDIL, a reduction in blood pressure generally occurs within two to five hours. During chronic administration, substantial blood pressure control lasts for 24 hours, with trough reductions in diastolic blood pressure approximately 40-50 percent of peak effects. The antihypertensive effect is dose-dependent and correlates with the plasma concentration of felodipine.

A reflex increase in heart rate frequently occurs during the first week of therapy; this increase attenuates over time. Heart rate increases of 5-10 beats per minute may be seen during chronic dosing. The increase is inhibited by beta-blocking agents.

The P-R interval of the ECG is not affected by felodipine when administered alone or in combination with a beta-blocking agent. Felodipine alone or in combination with a beta-blocking agent has been shown, in clinical and electrophysiologic studies, to have no significant effect on cardiac conduction (P-R, P-Q and H-V intervals).

In clinical trials in hypertensive patients without clinical evidence of left ventricular dysfunction, no symptoms suggestive of a negative inotropic effect were noted; however none would be expected in this population (see PRECAUTIONS).

Renal/Endocrine Effects

Renal vascular resistance is decreased by felodipine while glomerular filtration rate remains unchanged. Mild diuresis, natriuresis and kaliuresis have been observed during the first week of therapy. No significant effects on serum electrolytes were observed during short- and long-term therapy.

In clinical trials increases in plasma noradrenaline levels have been observed.

Clinical Studies

Felodipine produces dose-related decreases in systolic and diastolic blood pressure as demonstrated in six placebo-controlled, dose response studies using either immediate-release or extended-release dosage forms. These studies enrolled over 800 patients on active treatment, at total daily doses ranging from 2.5 to 20 mg. In those studies felodipine was administered either as monotherapy or was added to beta blockers. The results of the two studies with PLENDIL given once daily as monotherapy are shown in the table below:

MEAN REDUCTIONS IN BLOOD PRESSURE (mmHg)* Systolic/Diastolic				
Dose	N	Mean Peak Response	Mean Trough Response	Trough/Peak Ratios (%s)
Study 1 (8 weeks)				
2.5 mg	68	9.4/4.7	2.7/2.5	29/53
5 mg	69	9.5/6.3	2.4/3.7	25/59
10 mg	67	18.0/10.6	10.0/6.0	56/56
Study 2 (4 weeks)				
10 mg	50	5.3/7.2	1.5/3.2	33/40**
20 mg	50	11.3/10.2	4.5/3.2	43/34**

*Placebo response subtracted
**Different number of patients available for peak and trough measurements

INDICATIONS AND USAGE

PLENDIL is indicated for the treatment of hypertension. PLENDIL may be used alone or concomitantly with other antihypertensive agents.

CONTRAINDICATIONS

PLENDIL is contraindicated in patients who are hypersensitive to this product.

PRECAUTIONS

General

Hypotension: Felodipine, like other calcium antagonists, may occasionally precipitate significant hypotension and rarely syncope. It may lead to reflex tachycardia which in susceptible individuals may precipitate angina pectoris. (See ADVERSE REACTIONS.)

Heart Failure: Although acute hemodynamic studies in a small number of patients with NYHA Class II or III heart failure treated with felodipine have not demonstrated negative inotropic effects, safety in patients with heart failure has not been established. Caution therefore should be exercised when using PLENDIL in patients with heart failure or compromised ventricular function, particularly in combination with a beta blocker.

Elderly Patients or Patients with Impaired Liver Function: Patients over 65 years of age or patients with impaired liver function may have elevated plasma concentrations of felodipine and may therefore respond to lower doses of PLENDIL. These patients should have their blood pressure monitored closely during dosage adjustment of PLENDIL and should rarely require doses above 10 mg. (See CLINICAL PHARMACOLOGY and DOSAGE AND ADMINISTRATION.)

Peripheral Edema: Peripheral edema, generally mild and not associated with generalized fluid retention, was the most common adverse event in the clinical trials. The incidence of peripheral edema was both dose- and age-dependent. Frequency of peripheral edema ranged from about 10 percent in patients under 50 years of age taking 5 mg daily to about 30 percent in those over 60 years of age taking 20 mg daily. This adverse effect generally occurs within 2-3 weeks after the initiation of treatment.

Information for Patients

Patients should be instructed to take PLENDIL whole and not to crush or chew the tablets. They should be told that mild gingival hyperplasia (gum swelling) has been reported. Good dental hygiene decreases its incidence and severity.

NOTE: As with many other drugs, certain advice to patients being treated with PLENDIL is warranted. This information is intended to aid in the safe and effective use of this medication. It is not a disclosure of all possible adverse or intended effects.

Drug Interactions

Beta-Blocking Agents: A pharmacokinetic study of felodipine in conjunction with metoprolol demonstrated no significant effects on the pharmacokinetics of felodipine. The AUC and C_{max} of metoprolol, however, were increased approximately 31 and 38 percent, respectively. In controlled clinical trials, beta blockers including metoprolol were concurrently administered with felodipine and were well tolerated.

Cimetidine: In healthy subjects pharmacokinetic studies showed an approximately 50 percent increase in the area under the plasma concentration time curve (AUC) as well as the C_{max} of felodipine when given concomitantly with cimetidine. It is anticipated that a clinically significant interaction may occur in some hypertensive patients. Therefore, it is recommended that low doses of PLENDIL be used when given concomitantly with cimetidine.

Digoxin: When given concomitantly with felodipine the peak plasma concentration of digoxin was significantly increased. There was, however, no significant change in the AUC of digoxin.

Other Concomitant Therapy: In healthy subjects there were no clinically significant interac-

TABLETS
PLENDIL®
(FELODIPINE, MSD)
EXTENDED-RELEASE TABLETS

DESCRIPTION

PLENDIL* (Felodipine, MSD) is a calcium antagonist (calcium channel blocker). Felodipine is a dihydropyridine derivative that is chemically described as ± ethyl methyl 4-(2,3-dichlorophenyl)-1,4-dihydro-2,6-dimethyl-3,5-pyridine-dicarboxylate. Its empirical formula is $C_{18}H_{19}Cl_2NO_4$ and its structural formula is:

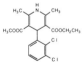

Felodipine is a slightly yellowish, crystalline powder with a molecular weight of 384.26. It is insoluble in water and is freely soluble in dichloromethane and ethanol. Felodipine is a racemic mixture.

Tablets PLENDIL provide extended release of felodipine. They are available as tablets containing 5 mg or 10 mg of felodipine for oral administration. In addition to the active ingredient felodipine, each tablet contains the following inactive ingredients: cellulose, iron oxides, lactose, polyethylene glycol, sodium stearyl fumarate, titanium dioxide and other ingredients.

CLINICAL PHARMACOLOGY

Mechanism of Action

Felodipine is a member of the dihydropyridine class of calcium channel antagonists (calcium channel blockers). It reversibly competes with nitrendipine and/or other calcium channel blockers for dihydropyridine binding sites, blocks voltage-dependent Ca^{++} currents in vascular smooth muscle and cultured rabbit atrial cells and blocks potassium-induced contracture of the rat portal vein.

In vitro studies show that the effects of felodipine on contractile processes are selective, with greater effects on vascular smooth muscle than cardiac muscle. Negative inotropic effects can be detected *in vitro*, but such effects have not been seen in intact animals.

The effect of felodipine on blood pressure is principally a consequence of a dose-related decrease of peripheral vascular resistance in man, with a modest reflex increase in heart rate (see *Cardiovascular Effects*). With the exception of a mild diuretic effect seen in several animal species and man, the effects of felodipine are accounted for by its effects on peripheral vascular resistance.

Pharmacokinetics and Metabolism

Following oral administration, felodipine is almost completely absorbed and undergoes extensive first-pass metabolism. The systemic bioavailability of PLENDIL is approximately 20 percent. Mean peak concentrations following the administration of PLENDIL are reached in 2.5 to 5 hours. Both peak plasma concentration and the area under the plasma concentration time curve (AUC) increase linearly with doses up to 20 mg. Felodipine is greater than 99 percent bound to plasma proteins.

Following intravenous administration, the plasma concentration of felodipine declined triexponentially with mean disposition half-lives of 4.8 minutes, 1.5 hours and 9.1 hours. The mean concentrations of the three individual

PLENDIL®
(Felodipine, MSD)
Extended-Release Tablets

phases to the overall AUC were 15, 40 and 45 percent, respectively, in the order of increasing $t_{\frac{1}{2}}$.

Following oral administration of the immediate-release formulation, the plasma level of felodipine also declined polyexponentially with a mean terminal $t_{\frac{1}{2}}$ of 11 to 16 hours. The mean peak and trough steady-state plasma concentrations achieved after 10 mg of the immediate-release formulation given once a day to normal volunteers, were 20 and 0.5 nmol/L, respectively. The trough plasma concentration of felodipine in most individuals was substantially below the concentration needed to effect a half-maximal decline in blood pressure (EC_{50}) [4-6 nmol/L for felodipine], thus precluding once a day dosing with the immediate-release formulation.

Following administration of a 10-mg dose of PLENDIL, the extended-release formulation, to young, healthy volunteers, mean peak and trough steady-state plasma concentrations of felodipine were 7 and 2 nmol/L, respectively. Corresponding values in hypertensive patients (mean age 64) after a 20-mg dose of PLENDIL were 23 and 7 nmol/L. Since the EC_{50} for felodipine is 4 to 6 nmol/L, a 5 to 10-mg dose of PLENDIL in some patients, and a 20-mg dose in others, would be expected to provide an antihypertensive effect that persists for 24 hours (see *Cardiovascular Effects* below and DOSAGE AND ADMINISTRATION).

The systemic plasma clearance of felodipine in young healthy subjects is about 0.8 L/min and the apparent volume of distribution is about 10 L/kg.

Following an oral or intravenous dose of ^{14}C-labeled felodipine in man, about 70 percent of the dose of radioactivity was recovered in urine and 10 percent in the feces. A negligible amount of intact felodipine is recovered in the urine and feces (<0.5%). Six metabolites, which account for 23 percent of the oral dose, have been identified; none has significant vasodilating activity.

Following administration of PLENDIL to hypertensive patients, mean peak plasma concentrations at steady state are about 20 percent higher than after a single dose. Blood pressure response is correlated with plasma concentrations of felodipine.

The bioavailability of PLENDIL is not influenced by the presence of food in the gastrointestinal tract. In a study of six patients, the bioavailability of felodipine was increased more than two-fold when taken with doubly concentrated grapefruit juice, compared to when taken with water or orange juice. A similar finding has been seen with some other dihydropyridine calcium antagonists, but to a lesser extent than that seen with felodipine.

Age Effects: Plasma concentrations of felodipine, after a single dose and at steady state, increase with age. Mean clearance of felodipine in elderly hypertensives (mean age 74) was only 45 percent of that of young volunteers (mean age 26). At steady state mean AUC for young patients was 39 percent of that for the elderly. Data for intermediate age ranges suggest that the AUCs fall between the extremes of the young and the elderly.

Hepatic Dysfunction: In patients with hepatic disease, the clearance of felodipine was reduced to about 60 percent of that seen in normal young volunteers.

Renal impairment does not alter the plasma concentration profile of felodipine; although higher concentrations of the metabolites are present in the plasma due to decreased urinary excretion, these are inactive.

tions when felodipine was given concomitantly with indomethacin or spironolactone.

Interaction with Food: See CLINICAL PHARMACOLOGY, *Pharmacokinetics and Metabolism.*

Carcinogenesis, Mutagenesis, Impairment of Fertility

In a two-year carcinogenicity study in rats fed felodipine at doses of 7.7, 23.1 or 69.3 mg/kg/day (up to 28 times* the maximum recommended human dose on a mg/m² basis), a dose-related increase in the incidence of benign interstitial cell tumors of the testes (Leydig cell tumors) was observed in treated male rats. These tumors were not observed in a similar study in mice at doses up to 138.6 mg/kg/day (28 times* the maximum recommended human dose on a mg/m² basis). Felodipine, at the doses employed in the two-year rat study, has been shown to lower testicular testosterone and to produce a corresponding increase in serum luteinizing hormone in rats. The Leydig cell tumor development is possibly secondary to these hormonal effects which have not been observed in man.

In this same rat study a dose-related increase in the incidence of focal squamous cell hyperplasia compared to control was observed in the esophageal groove of male and female rats in all dose groups. No other drug-related esophageal or gastric pathology was observed in the rats or with chronic administration in mice and dogs. The latter species, like man, has no anatomical structure comparable to the esophageal groove.

Felodipine was not carcinogenic when fed to mice at doses of up to 138.6 mg/kg/day (28 times* the maximum recommended human dose on a mg/m² basis) for periods of up to 80 weeks in males and 99 weeks in females.

Felodipine did not display any mutagenic activity *in vitro* in the Ames microbial mutagenicity test or in the mouse lymphoma forward mutation assay. No clastogenic potential was seen *in vivo* in the mouse micronucleus test at oral doses up to 2500 mg/kg (506 times* the maximum recommended human dose on a mg/m² basis) or *in vitro* in a human lymphocyte chromosome aberration assay.

A fertility study in which male and female rats were administered doses of 3.8, 9.6 or 26.9 mg/kg/day showed no significant effect of felodipine on reproductive performance.

Pregnancy

Pregnancy Category C

Teratogenic Effects: Studies in pregnant rabbits administered doses of 0.46, 1.2, 2.3 and 4.6 mg/kg/day (from 0.4 to 4 times* the maximum recommended human dose on a mg/m² basis) showed digital anomalies consisting of reduction in size and degree of ossification of the terminal phalanges in the fetuses. The frequency and severity of the changes appeared dose-related and were noted even at the lowest dose. These changes have been shown to occur with other members of the dihydropyridine class and are possibly a result of compromised uterine blood flow. Similar fetal anomalies were not observed in rats given felodipine.

In a teratology study in cynomolgus monkeys no reduction in the size of the terminal phalanges was observed but an abnormal position of the distal phalanges was noted in about 40 percent of the fetuses.

Nonteratogenic Effects: A prolongation of parturition with difficult labor and an increased frequency of fetal and early postnatal deaths were observed in rats administered doses of 9.6

*Based on patient weight of 50 kg

mg/kg/day (4 times* the maximum human dose on a mg/m² basis) and above.

Significant enlargement of the mammary glands in excess of the normal enlargement for pregnant rabbits was found with doses greater than or equal to 1.2 mg/kg/day (equal to the maximum human dose on a mg/m² basis). This effect occurred only in pregnant rabbits and regressed during lactation. Similar changes in the mammary glands were not observed in rats or monkeys.

There are no adequate and well-controlled studies in pregnant women. If felodipine is used during pregnancy, or if the patient becomes pregnant while taking this drug, she should be apprised of the potential hazard to the fetus, possible digital anomalies of the infant, and the potential effects of felodipine on labor and delivery, and on the mammary glands of pregnant females.

Nursing Mothers

It is not known whether this drug is secreted in human milk and because of the potential for serious adverse reactions from felodipine in the infant, a decision should be made whether to discontinue nursing or to discontinue the drug, taking into account the importance of the drug to the mother.

Pediatric Use

Safety and effectiveness in children have not been established.

ADVERSE REACTIONS

In controlled studies in the United States and overseas approximately 3000 patients were treated with felodipine as either the extended-release or the immediate-release formulation.

The most common clinical adverse experiences reported with PLENDIL administered as monotherapy in all settings and with all dosage forms of felodipine were peripheral edema and headache. Peripheral edema was generally mild, but it was age- and dose-related and resulted in discontinuation of therapy in about 4 percent of the enrolled patients. Discontinuation of therapy due to any clinical adverse experience occurred in about 9 percent of the patients receiving PLENDIL, principally for peripheral edema, headache, or flushing.

Adverse experiences that occurred with an incidence of 1.5 percent or greater during monotherapy with PLENDIL without regard to causality are compared to placebo in the table below.

Percent of Patients with Adverse Effects in Controlled Trials of PLENDIL as Monotherapy
(Incidence of discontinuations shown in parentheses)

Adverse Effect	PLENDIL % N = 730		Placebo % N = 283
Peripheral Edema	22.3	(4.2)	3.5
Headache	18.6	(2.1)	10.6
Flushing	6.4	(1.0)	1.1
Dizziness	5.8	(0.8)	3.2
Upper Respiratory Infection	5.5	(0.1)	1.1
Asthenia	4.7	(0.1)	2.8
Cough	2.9	(0.0)	0.4
Paresthesia	2.5	(0.1)	1.8
Dyspepsia	2.3	(0.0)	1.4
Chest Pain	2.1	(0.1)	1.4
Nausea	1.9	(0.8)	1.1
Muscle Cramps	1.9	(0.0)	1.1
Palpitation	1.8	(0.5)	2.5
Abdominal Pain	1.8	(0.3)	1.1
Constipation	1.6	(0.1)	1.1
Diarrhea	1.6	(0.1)	1.1
Pharyngitis	1.6	(0.0)	0.4
Rhinorrhea	1.6	(0.0)	0.0
Back Pain	1.6	(0.0)	1.1
Rash	1.5	(0.1)	1.1

*Based on patient weight of 50 kg

PLENDIL®
(Felodipine, MSD)
Extended-Release Tablets

3

In the two dose response studies using PLENDIL as monotherapy, the following table describes the incidence (percent) of adverse experiences that were dose-related:

Adverse Effect	Placebo N = 121	2.5 mg N = 71	5.0 mg N = 72	10.0 mg N = 123	20 mg N = 50
Peripheral Edema	2.5	1.4	13.9	19.5	36.0
Palpitation	0.8	1.4	0.0	2.4	12.0
Headache	12.4	11.3	11.1	18.7	28.0
Flushing	0.0	4.2	2.8	8.1	20.0

In addition, adverse experiences that occurred in 0.5 up to 1.5 percent of patients who received PLENDIL in all controlled clinical studies (listed in order of decreasing severity within each category) and serious adverse events that occurred at a lower rate or were found during marketing experience (those lower rate events are in italics) were: *Body as a Whole:* Facial edema, warm sensation; *Cardiovascular:* Tachycardia, *myocardial infarction, hypotension, syncope, angina pectoris,* arrhythmia; *Digestive:* Vomiting, dry mouth, flatulence; *Hematologic: Anemia; Musculoskeletal:* Arthralgia, arm pain, knee pain, leg pain, foot pain, hip pain, myalgia; *Nervous/Psychiatric:* Depression, anxiety disorders, insomnia, irritability, nervousness, somnolence; *Respiratory:* Bronchitis, influenza, sinusitis, dyspnea, epistaxis, respiratory infection, sneezing; *Skin:* Contusion, erythema, urticaria; *Urogenital:* Decreased libido, impotence, urinary frequency, urinary urgency, dysuria.

Felodipine, as an immediate release formulation, has also been studied as monotherapy in 680 patients with hypertension in U.S. and overseas controlled clinical studies. Other adverse experiences not listed above and with an incidence of 0.5 percent or greater include: *Body as a Whole:* Fatigue; *Digestive:* Gastrointestinal pain; *Musculoskeletal:* Arthritis, local weakness, neck pain, shoulder pain, ankle pain; *Nervous/Psychiatric:* Tremor; *Respiratory:* Rhinitis; *Skin:* Hyperhidrosis, pruritus; *Special Senses:* Blurred vision, tinnitus; *Urogenital:* Nocturia.

Gingival Hyperplasia: Gingival hyperplasia, usually mild, occurred in <0.5 percent of patients in controlled studies. This condition may be avoided or may regress with improved dental hygiene. (See PRECAUTIONS, *Information for Patients.*)

Clinical Laboratory Test Findings
Serum Electrolytes: No significant effects on serum electrolytes were observed during short- and long-term therapy (see CLINICAL PHARMACOLOGY, *Renal/Endocrine Effects*).

Serum Glucose: No significant effects on fasting serum glucose were observed in patients treated with PLENDIL in the U.S. controlled study.

Liver Enzymes: One of two episodes of elevated serum transaminases decreased once drug was discontinued in clinical studies; no follow-up was available for the other patient.

OVERDOSAGE

Oral doses of 240 mg/kg in male and female mice, respectively and 2390 mg/kg and 2250 mg/kg in male and female rats, respectively, caused significant lethality.

In a suicide attempt, one patient took 150 mg felodipine together with 15 tablets each of atenolol and spironolactone and 20 tablets of nitrazepam. The patient's blood pressure and heart rate were normal on admission to hospital; he subsequently recovered without significant sequelae.

Overdosage might be expected to cause excessive peripheral vasodilation with marked hypotension and possibly bradycardia.

If severe hypotension occurs, symptomatic treatment should be instituted. The patient should be placed supine with the legs elevated. The administration of intravenous fluids may be useful to treat hypotension due to overdosage with calcium antagonists. In case of accompanying bradycardia, atropine (0.5-1 mg) should be administered intravenously. Sympathomimetic drugs may also be given if the physician feels they are warranted.

It has not been established whether felodipine can be removed from the circulation by hemodialysis.

DOSAGE AND ADMINISTRATION

The recommended initial dose is 5 mg once a day. Therapy should be adjusted individually according to patient response, generally at intervals of not less than two weeks. The usual dosage range is 5-10 mg once daily. The maximum recommended daily dose is 20 mg once a day. That dose in clinical trials showed an increased blood pressure response but a large increase in the rate of peripheral edema and other vasodilatory adverse events (see ADVERSE REACTIONS). Modification of the recommended dosage is usually not required in patients with renal impairment.

PLENDIL should be swallowed whole and not crushed or chewed.

Use in the Elderly or Patients with Impaired Liver Function: Patients over 65 years of age or patients with impaired liver function, because they may develop higher plasma concentrations of felodipine, should have their blood pressure monitored closely during dosage adjustment (see PRECAUTIONS). In general, doses above 10 mg should not be considered in these patients.

HOW SUPPLIED

No. 3585 — Tablets PLENDIL, 5 mg, are light red-brown, round convex tablets, with code MSD 451 on one side and PLENDIL on the other. They are supplied as follows:
NDC 0006-0451-28 unit dose packages of 100
NDC 0006-0451-58 unit of use bottles of 100
NDC 0006-0451-31 unit of use bottles of 30.
No. 3586 — Tablets PLENDIL, 10 mg, are red-brown, round convex tablets, with code MSD 452 on one side and PLENDIL on the other. They are supplied as follows:
NDC 0006-0452-28 unit dose packages of 100
NDC 0006-0452-58 unit of use bottles of 100
NDC 0006-0452-31 unit of use bottles of 30.
Storage
Store below 30°C (86°F). Keep container tightly closed. Protect from light.

MERCK SHARP & DOHME, Division of Merck & Co., Inc.
West Point, Pa. 19486

MSD
MERCK
SHARP &
DOHME

Printed in USA

A.H.F.S. Category: 24:04

Issued July 1991   DC7650202

4